POLARITY THERAPY

where ENERGY meets
STRUCTURE and FUNCTION

Phil Young PTP

Masterworks International Publishing

Published in Great Britain 2017 by

MASTERWORKS INTERNATIONAL

27 Old Gloucester Street

London

WC1N 3XX

England

Tel: 00353 (0)86 325 2645

Email: admin@mwipublishing.com

Web: http://www.mwipublishing.com

Cover design by MWI design. Graphics: 1. Sd render medical illustration of the human spine © Maya - dreamstime.com. 2. Spine - dreamstime.com 3. Energy Grid © Morag Campbell

13 digit ISBN: 978-0-9933465-2-1

This book is a revised, expanded and updated version of the book "The Art of Polarity Therapy, A Practitioner's Perspective," published by Prism Press UK, 1990.

Printed in the UK/USA by Lightning Source

CONTENTS

Polarity Therapy balances and stimulates the body's life energy currents. It does not treat or diagnose illness or disease. It is not intended to be a substitute for needed medical care.

Introduction to the New Edition

This is a book of two voices, both mine, but one from today and the other from over 27 years ago. Remarkably, in the process of revising the original book, I found that I agreed with more or less everything in it. I still teach all of this material in my courses. The primary difference between my early voice and my current voice is the greater depth of understanding and insight that I now have. You can hear this most clearly in the major expansion of the chapter on Structural Balancing. In the original book the theoretical exposition was a mere 3000 words. In this new edition, it is nearly 10 times as long.

The other chapters that have been majorly revised and expanded are those on the Five Elements and Self Help. The theoretical underpinnings of all the bodywork techniques have been expanded. Throughout the rest of the book I have changed little, beyond updating time-sensitive references.

This book was originally designed to be a companion book to Polarity Therapy - The Power that Heals by my teacher Alan Siegel, MS, ND. Alan's book was republished in a revised and expanded form in 2006 and re-titled Polarity Therapy - Healing with Life Energy. Both of these new, revised editions still complement each other.

Over the last 30 years of teaching Polarity Therapy, I have been aware that students follow two major routes into the art. One mimics Dr. Stone's own journey, which was from being an osteopath and chiropractor whose clinical experience forced him into re-evaluating the role of energy in the healing process. The other path is when a student of one or more of the wide variety of healing modalities, ranging from aromatherapy to reflexology or any of the multitude of energy-based approaches, feels the need for a more complete approach to therapeutic change. My own journey was the latter, but my experience of working with students of the former path, those who followed directly in Dr. Stone's footsteps, led me more and more deeply into the osteopathic underpinnings of Polarity Therapy. As you will realise when you study this book, I have enjoyed that journey immensely. It is my hope that you will feel as inspired as I do by the fruits of that 30-year-long process.

Phil Young, PTP, Ireland, 2017

phily@masterworksinternational.com

Introduction to the 1st Edition

This book is in part a very personal statement concerning my own approach to Polarity Therapy as a full-time practitioner and is also a very clear, concise guide to the many techniques that were not included in *Polarity Therapy, the Power that Heals* written by my teacher Alan Siegel N.D. and myself. If you have not read that book it would be helpful if you did, as it will make this one more accessible, though anyone with a good basic understanding of Polarity Therapy will find this book an invaluable guide to using this fascinating healing art at a professional level. I have structured the book rather like a Polarity session beginning with the preliminaries, taking the case history, on through the diagnosis, the energy balancing bodywork and finally reviewing the whole process.

It is a distillation of the knowledge and insight that I have gained since becoming a practicing therapist. During this time I have given many thousands of treatments to clients with problems ranging from low back pain to advanced cancerous conditions. For the last three years I have also been running a successful professional training programme in England covering all aspects of Polarity Therapy. I have also, like most other Polarity therapists, spent many a fascinating hour poring over the information-packed, but ultimately confusing books written by the founder of Polarity Therapy Dr. Randolph Stone. I truly hope this book is a little clearer. I urge you not to give up reading the original books as they contain the experience of many decades of healing work. A level of experience that I cannot match, yet!

At this time (1989) there is a big movement worldwide to establish minimum standards of excellence in the practice of Polarity Therapy, a move that I heartily applaud and am directly involved in. As Moshe Feldenkrais, the late originator of an amazing technique of movement re-education pointed out before his death, there is no system that has been developed in the realm of somatics that has not been improved upon by the students and practitioners of the system in the following years after the passing of the founder. A sentiment that I am sure Dr. Stone and his named successor Pierre Pannetier would share. Do not be afraid to be creative in your practice. One has only to read Dr. Stone's books to realize that he was a true eclectic who took different parts of many healing arts and blended this knowledge with his own practical experience and unique insight to create Polarity Therapy.

I hope you enjoy studying and applying in your own practice the techniques and insights that I offer in this book and find them as useful as I have. Happy polarizing!

1. First Thoughts

In essence all therapy is about creating a relationship with the client that is supportive enough to give them the confidence to heal themselves. All relationships are about contact, communication and change. It has been said that the whole course of a relationship can be charted from the first five minutes of contact between the people involved. If this is true, then in the case of Polarity Therapy the first few minutes of contact with a client occur most frequently over the telephone. It is important to have some awareness of how to deal with the kind of questions that are raised and to have an ability to present yourself and your work in an appropriate light. The most frequently asked questions are: what is Polarity Therapy? how does it work? can it help me? how long will it be before I get better? does it work for everyone? are you qualified? There are many other questions that you will be asked but these are the main recurring ones. These questions are often asked during the first actual session, particularly if the issues they concern have not been dealt with in the very first contact. Indeed it is possible to set your practice up in such a way that these issues are only dealt with during the first face-to-face contact, either the first session or during a specific interview created to deal with them. An informatory interview is a particularly good idea if you feel uncomfortable on the telephone.

As a practitioner of Polarity Therapy do you actually know what you want to achieve in a series of sessions? Is your work orientated towards personal growth, or do you view it as an alternative to allopathic medicine? Do you practice preventative health care and maintenance, or healing in which your hands and energy are superior substitutes for modem drug therapy? Do you do both? Perhaps you see Polarity as relaxation therapy for stress release. I can see some purists throwing up their hands in horror at such a thought, yet if some 80 per cent of all illness is caused by stress (a figure which I have noticed goes up every year!) such an approach to Polarity Therapy can hardly be glibly dismissed. Do you practice it as a form of postural and movement therapy? It is obviously true to say that there is an enormous diversity in the approaches to treatment that a Polarity practitioner can offer. The main thing is to know what you do and be able to articulate it in a clear, precise fashion.

In your first contact with a client it is important to communicate with them in terms that they can understand and relate to easily. There is no point in talking about chakras, life energy and the five elements if these terms are not part of the client's vocabulary. There is a need to educate but do not try to begin by getting into deep involved expositions on energy. Develop some very simple explanations about the nature of Polarity Therapy around terminology that you know everyone is likely to understand, perhaps using such terms as stress, relaxation, good circulation, nervous system stimulation and so on. If you want to talk about energy you can use analogies about flat batteries, magnetism, electrical generating stations, and the national grid. Always begin by speaking to clients in a language they can understand, to create a rapport, then you can start to teach them a new one. To create a secure relationship with a client it is vitally important that they feel they understand the nature of the therapeutic process. It is not important that the explanation you give them is completely accurate, just that it allows them to feel safe, secure and confident.

In some systems of alternative medicine the practitioners are recommended, by the various training establishments, to wear white jackets or some other type of uniform whilst giving treatments. I can see why this might have practical value in some therapies but I have always felt that most of my clients were trying to get away from people who wear white coats or uniforms. The clothing you wear whilst giving sessions can have a profound effect on your client. In fact, the colour alone could become a form of therapeutic intervention, provided that you have an understanding of the effects of colour upon consciousness and the life energy. If you are going to teach Polarity Yoga as part of your sessions then your clothing obviously needs to be loose and comfortable, which is fine as long as you know in advance that you intend to do this, but what if it suddenly seems appropriate and you are wearing tight trousers? I finally came to the conclusion that it is important to wear clothing that is comfortable, loose, and smart enough to do anything I wanted to in. I frequently find it useful to put one knee on the bodywork table for support when giving a session and some clothing just does not allow you to do this with dignity—an even greater problem for female practitioners who may be wearing dresses or skirts.

The room you practice in, its decor and ambience can also have a profound effect on your clients. It is ideal if you can set aside a room that is used only for giving treatments. This allows a certain quality of energy to build up in it that is highly beneficial to the healing process. If you have to use a room that is used for other purposes as well, then develop a few simple ways of changing its ambience by doing something other than just setting up a bodywork table. Burn some incense, put up a few charts, whatever will make you feel that it is now a treatment room and not your living room or den. From the client's perspective it will make the whole therapeutic experience more professional, and that is important, certainly in the beginning stages of therapy. At a later date when the relationship is more familiar a relaxed approach is also valuable, as it helps to get away from the 'therapist as god' syndrome that is sometimes cultivated by practitioners, a scenario that is ultimately destructive and de-humanizing in my opinion.

When giving a Polarity session it has been said that the client should remove all jewellery as the metal has its own effect on the client's energy field; an effect that may be in opposition to the balance you are trying to create in a session. Dr. Stone pointed out many times the powerful effect that gold and silver have on the energy fields, and indeed used these metals extensively in his own practice. I never ask a client to take rings off before a session precisely because of the effect of gold and silver on the life energy. I believe that if the effect of these metals is as potent as Dr. Stone indicated, when a client puts the rings back on at the end of the session there will be an instant distortion of the balance that I have so carefully created. I know from my own experience that it is possible to create good balance and flow of life energy when a client is still wearing their jewellery, and that it will not then be a factor that could disrupt the balance that has been achieved after the session. In some cases because of acute energetic sensitivity in general, I have felt it necessary to advise a client to stop wearing jewellery altogether.

The amount of metal in a bodywork table can also have a significant effect on your energy balancing work, so the less the better. I also know from my own experience that there is a powerful energy field that emanates from the kind of wood used in a table's construction. I myself once asked a master woodworker to create a bodywork table for me, and finally chose beech as the dominant wood in its structure because having scanned many different kinds of wood I felt happiest with its energy quality, although its weight meant that the table is not portable. I am not saying that beech is *the* wood out of which to make a Polarity table but it is the one that suits me best. You may feel differently. It is certainly an area worth exploring if you can, but do not get worried about it if you are not able. Simply get a table you really like even if it is metal and marine plywood. Your positive thoughts will more than compensate. The width of a table is also important, 30 inches (76 cm) wide being a minimum. This can be a problem, particularly in some countries, where if you are a massage therapist who has trained in Polarity Therapy at a later date, you will probably already have a table, and standard massage tables are usually only 24-26 inches (60-66 cm) wide. You need a table wide enough to allow a client's arms to rest fully relaxed at their sides.

In Polarity Therapy there is a great deal of discussion given to the idea that the practitioner should be 'neutral' when working with clients. What does this actually mean?

My own teacher emphasized that because everybody heals at different rates, it was important not to expect to see instant physical results after doing a manipulation as your criteria for success. Pierre Pannetier used to say that we as practitioners do not do anything, it is the life energy that does it all. Pierre also told students to remember that 'You are not the healer.' To me this meant that I did not need to become attached to the results of my treatments. If they worked, that was fine, and if they did not then that was also fine. However, it did seem to me after practicing for some time that whilst this had a great deal of benefit for me in that it meant effectively that I never failed regardless of whether a client changed or not, and allowed me to maintain positive feelings concerning my therapeutic skill particularly as this position never called my skills into question, I began to see it as being something less than desirable. I actually became a therapist to facilitate people's self-healing processes, so to adopt a position of neutrality in relation to treatment somehow did not give me a basis upon which to evaluate how good I was. I have always maintained that most, if not all, practitioners of any healing art do it because when they are able to help a client move towards wholeness their egos are given a powerful boost (and their bank balance does not suffer either). There is often a great deal of self deception about why anyone should want to practice as a therapist. When I began to look at my motivations as clearly and honestly as I could, I realized that I did not want to practice from a neutral position, not least because it denied me a certain level of ego satisfaction. I would question any statements from a practitioner to the effect that they did not experience any ego satisfaction from their work, that they only practiced for higher or more noble reasons. I myself am a therapist for both selfless, loving, spiritual reasons and much more pragmatic, ego and material needs.

To facilitate the expression of all my reasons for being a therapist, I began to adopt a position in relation to my work that I call 'balanced positive' as opposed to neutral. In effect, what this means is that I approach Polarity Therapy with the belief that I am sufficiently skilful to be able to resolve even the most complicated life problems for the client, that I do not expect to see instantaneous healing, but I acknowledge that it can and does occur, so that if a change does not occur for the client I will not consider it a failure on my part, the client's or the life energy. I will look at it as an opportunity to ascertain in what areas I need to expand my knowledge and skills. It is true that the life energy does everything, but it can only do so when it is flowing freely. My job as a therapist is to make it possible for the life energy to do the healing, and I have found that for me a balanced positive attitude creates the greatest possibility of this occurring. My intention is an extremely powerful, direct yet balanced desire for the client to be able to resolve his problems. An intention that allows me to effect rapid and profound changes in their energy fields.

In Chinese energy theory a great deal of importance is attached to the concept of 'i' and its relationship to 'chi,' the Chinese term for life or breath energy. The translation of the Chinese word 'i' is 'mind,' 'intent,' or sometimes 'mind intent.' The relationship between these two concepts is often expressed as the 'chi' (or energy) flows at the behest of the 'i' or mind intent. To put it another way, your intention, the pattern of your thinking, can control the movement of life energy in your body. It is this law that is fundamental to the effectiveness of nearly all self-healing visualizations and affirmations. As Polarity therapists this fact has enormous significance in that it is your mind intent, or to put it more simply your intention, that controls the quality and kind of energetic interaction that occurs between you and your client.

The greater the clarity of thought and intention that you bring to your sessions the more effective your treatments will become. When I began practicing Polarity Therapy one of the first things that I became interested in was whether I was sufficiently sensitive to be able to differentiate between the different elemental energies in a client's energy field. At first I did feel that I was able to tell which quality of energy I was interacting with at any time. Then I began to notice that if I had evaluated a client as having a particular kind of elemental imbalance, then that was always the quality of energy that I interacted with during the bodywork. Quite frankly after a while I really began to wonder how it was that I always seemed to get it right! How was I always able to deduce before a treatment began what elements were out of balance? Particularly when some of the treatments did not create any significant change in the client's condition. Most obviously I was not always right! I then began to experiment with making clearly false-to-fact evaluations concerning the particular energetic imbalances that a client was manifesting, and working on that basis. I worked in the full belief that the evaluation that I made was the correct one. What happened was that the energy I predominantly interacted with was always the one that I had falsely decided to be the problem. It began to seem more and more that the concept that energy follows thought was true not just in terms of controlling your own energy flows and in the process of self healing, but it also applied in my interaction with the client's energy. These and other experiences showed me just how powerful a practitioner's intention is in determining both the quality and function of their energy release work.

Qualities of Touch

In Polarity Therapy the most active way of communicating with the client is through physical touch or, more correctly, energetic touch. Dr. Stone defined three types of touch that can be used in Polarity Therapy. To use the Sanskrit terminology they are Rajasic, Satvic, and Tamasic. Roughly translated these types of touch could be called, respectively: stimulating, balancing and dispersing. Historically, there has always been something of a split or schism amongst practitioners of Polarity Therapy concerning the relative value of the tamasic quality of touch. However, before we look at this in more detail a deeper look at each kind of touch as defined by Dr. Stone is appropriate.

Rajasic

The function of rajasic or stimulating touch is to move energy. To stir it up. It is done with a positive but light hand contact that moulds itself to the contours of the body. The hand is then vibrated, moved backwards and forwards or in circular fashion, so that the movement which occurs is the skin moving over the underlying tissue. In other words, the hand does not slide over the skin but stays in the same place. Depending on the amplitude and range of your movement the client's body may go into oscillation, a gentle rocking motion. This kind of touch resonates with the outward or centrifugal movement of energy in the client's body, the energy flow as it moves from the core of the energy field to the circumference. It is a positively charged contact.

Satvic

The function of satvic or balancing touch is to calm the energy, to bring it into balance, to smooth its flow so that there is no turbulence. It is done with a very light touch that moulds itself gently to the contour of the body. There is no intentional physical movement involved. This kind of touch resonates with all the neutrally charged areas of the body, the central axes, and the areas where the energy currents cross over creating perfect balance, specifically the chakras and the joints. It is a neutrally charged contact.

Tamasic

The function of the tamasic or dispersing touch is to break up chronic energy blocks within the body's energy field. It is done with a deep penetrating touch that goes down into the underlying tissues beneath the contact area. It is a deep tissue technique that seeks to release the energy locked in areas of extreme muscular tension, areas where the physical tension is impeding the flow of energy, blood, lymph and nutrients, where there is a lot of accumulated toxicity and poor drainage. It releases energy so that it can complete its return flow from the circumference back to the core of the energy field, the centripetal flow of energy. It is a negatively charged contact.

All Polarity therapists use the rajasic and satvic touches, but only some use the tamasic touch as well. Pierre Pannetier, the successor to Dr. Stone, emphasized the lighter rajasic and satvic work on the basis that people in pain are already hurting enough, so what justification was there for adding to it? Since the mid 1990s the influence of cranial work on the practice of Polarity Therapy has inclined many practitioners to focus on lighter satvic touch in their work, more or less excluding rajasic and tamasic touch.

Dr. Stone says in his writings that patients do not easily forgive you for inflicting pain on them, and that when giving a treatment you should be gentle. He also recommends deep work and heavy pressure release. If we look at the basis of his reasoning for using a deep tamasic touch it is in essence that a blockage manifesting as a congestion in the muscle tissue indicates a lack of circulation, and that the key to releasing this is to drain the muscle of toxins and fluids by deep pressure which will squeeze the stagnant fluids out, creating a vacuum effect, a space that will be filled by fresh blood and prana that will facilitate the detoxification process. Energetically it is also true that opposites attract in the centripetal flow of energy and that like charges repel, so by using a negatively charged touch on a blocked area with a negative charge, there is a repelling effect that will push the blocked energy back to its source, releasing the flow. This process almost always induces real soreness for a period of time until the last of the toxins are cleared, all of which is indicative of the energy currents moving again. This I know through my own experimentation with tamasic touch to be perfectly valid. However, I have also discovered that it is not necessary. It is quite possible to release these stagnant areas by using the rajasic touch and even the satvic touch as defined by Dr. Stone.

Dr. Stone says in his writings that the key to releasing blockages at the congested negative poles is 'stimulation.' The tamasic work is extremely stimulating and creates very fast results and a lot of discomfort. The rajasic touch is also stimulating. The key to making it effective on very congested areas is to find the right direction of application that releases the energy. The end result is the same. The toxins are cleared and the energy flows freely again, but the difference is that it takes a little longer and it is a lot less painful. The time difference, in my experience, is that if a tamasic treatment is going to clear the system it takes between twenty- four and forty-eight hours, whereas a rajasic treatment will take some two to four days, a totally negligible difference in my opinion. There is also a possibility that if you release too much toxicity into the client's system all at once, that this can create secondary problems if their eliminative system is already overloaded. This is a serious point that you should consider in all your work, particularly if you are working with cancerous conditions. It is quite possible to break up tumors using energy-based techniques, Polarity or otherwise. Always make sure the eliminative system is functioning well enough to deal with the massive amount of debris that can be dumped into the system during the healing process.

It is also possible to release deep congestion with satvic touch. This can be done in two ways. Firstly, using the fact that life energy flows from your right to your left hand, you can easily bring increasing amounts of energy into the blocked area by placing your left hand on it and having your right hand on the positive pole of the particular area, and waiting until you feel the energy reacting very strongly beneath your left hand. Once this is happening simply reverse your hands and send the energy back to its supply pole, the positive pole. You have now created a powerful complete flow of life energy through the blocked area, which will clear the congestion. It is also possible to extend this technique to include the negative pole of the blocked area.

The other way, which simply involves holding the blocked area, is based upon the fact that the polarity of these deeply blocked areas is negative and that it is the inward or return flow of energy that is blocked. In this phase of energy movement 'opposites attract,' and as a satvic touch is in effect an opposite charge to the blocked area (remember that positive and negative are relative terms, so a neutrally charged touch is still positive in relation to a blocked area that is negatively charged), you will in effect attract the energy block towards your contact hand, regardless of whether it is your right or left hand, as long as it is acting as a satvic neutrally charged contact. As you move the blockage out of its original position, fresh prana will instantly begin to flow in and through that area again. At the moment the energy block, the stagnant prana, moves it has to break up and disperse because its static nature has changed. It is moving again, and if it is moving it is no longer by definition blocked energy, so it has to disperse back into the overall economy of the body's energy field. This particular energetic process also occurs when using rajasic touch because of the polarities involved. In terms of the time these satvic releases take to work, in my experience, they seem to follow some logic all of their own. Sometimes the change seems almost instantaneous even with physical tension, and at other times it takes four or five days. I have never been able to discover a discernible pattern.

Some practitioners have expressed the opinion that the 'light' work is too slow, but I have never been able to get a satisfactory answer as to how they define 'slow' in relation to energy work as being a pejorative. I hardly think that the difference of a few days or even a couple of weeks, can be thought of as a valid objection to the effectiveness of the light work. From the client's point of view the main consideration is often quick relief from pain. The rajasic and satvic work is no less effective than the tamasic work in this area in relation to time, as there is always a significant reduction in pain immediately. It is the full resolution that just takes that much longer. In fact, I have some doubts that a full resolution ever truly occurs when the tamasic work is used extensively. My own personal experience of working on clients who have been treated by practitioners whose approach uses a lot of deep tamasic work, is that the energy blocks are often pushed deeper into the system. What has happened is that as I have worked gently on areas that have apparently been resolved of energetic disturbance by other practitioners, the original problem has reappeared in full force. To me this indicates a deep suppression of the imbalance as opposed to a proper resolution. I can from my own personal experience of tamasic work see how this might occur, in that if pain is indicative of blocked energy, and if energetically there is a contraction in any problem area, then increasing the pain by deep work can simply cause greater contraction at a deeper level. It also seems possible that it may cause the blockage to be pushed so deep that it enters into the mind energy field and becomes, to use Dr. Stone's terminology, a sensory energy block.

You have only to experience deep tamasic work on yourself to realize the degree of mental-emotional withdrawal that is a natural response to the pain it creates. As energy follows thought this is the last thing you want to occur when trying to resolve disturbances in the energy fields. Encouraging the client to go into the pain rather than withdraw from it is a useful technique to use when doing tamasic work, but unfortunately unless the client has a high degree of masochism in their makeup they will only go into the pain with a portion of their conscious awareness. A full release can only occur when both conscious and unconscious awareness is involved totally. As one of the functions of the unconscious mind is protection, then even though there may be a conscious sense of going into the pain, the unconscious is quite likely to be watching the therapist and saying something internally like 'what do you think I am, stupid or something? You are the one causing most of the pain, and you want me to experience it more!.'

As a descriptive metaphor let us look at water and its behaviour as a good analogy for energetic processes. In any blocked area we could typify the blockages as being ice. To allow the water to flow freely the ice must be removed. This could be done in one of two

17

ways: either tamasically by hitting it and breaking it up, or rajasic / satvically by melting it with the heat of your hands. In the former the ice will certainly break up, allowing the water to flow again, but what about the shards of ice that would get smashed into the surrounding structure in the process? What about the damage caused to the surrounding structure by the original impact? What about the fragments that are released? Perhaps some are still too big to break up naturally and flow freely through the whole system, necessitating your having to follow them around breaking them up when they get stuck. A time consuming process! Whereas, in the latter case, the icy blockage just melts, becoming water again and allowing free flow with no damage to the surrounding area and no likelihood of it causing a blockage elsewhere. I know the scenario I would prefer to create if this analogy has any validity.

Before moving on from our exploration of the three' classic' kinds of Polarity contacts, as defined by Dr. Stone, if we go back to his definitions of the different kinds of touch it is obvious that there is both a physical component to each touch and an energetic component. It is possible to create at least nine different kinds of touch by combining these components in different ways. The physical component of rajasic touch is a firm surface contact that moves tissues beneath the skin. Satvic touch is very light surface contact only, with little or no movement. Tamasic touch is deep sub-surface contact achieved by strong pressure, and can be done with or without movement. As movement is a variable quality in each kind of touch, leaving it aside as a consideration the physical parameters we are left with are contacts that are surface, just below surface and deep into the structure. The energetic component of rajasic touch is its positive charge that increases the outflow of energy, of satvic touch it is its neutral charge that balances, and of tamasic touch it is its negative charge that sends the currents back to their source. Dr. Stone typified the positive outflow of energy as warm and creative, the negative inflow as cool and constructive, and the neuter source and its reflection at the most expansive point of the outflow (and beginning of the inflow) as stillness. Energetically I like to think that the positive charged touch says 'let's go and play,' the neutral charged touch says 'let's rest and relax awhile,' and the negatively charged touch says 'let's go home.' I used these and other relevant images as ways of attuning my conscious intention to arouse the energy currents as specifically as possible.

This gives the possibility of nine different types of touch, as set out opposite, all creating quite different effects.

	PHYSICAL	ENERGETIC
1.	Surface Touch	Neutral Charge
2.	Below Surface	Neutral Charge
3.	Deep Touch	Neutral Charge
4.	Surface Touch	Positive Charge
5.	Below Surface	Positive Charge
6.	Deep Touch	Positive Charge
7.	Surface Touch	Negative Charge
8.	Below Surface	Negative Charge
9.	Deep Touch	Negative Charge

Physical movement or lack of it could be added to the model, creating further permutations. The classic rajasic touch would be a no. 5 type touch, the satvic contact a no.1 type touch, and the tamasic contact a no. 9 type touch. It is clear that there is a way of modulating the classical tamasic contact so that you can clear congested tissues but without undue pain, and also that you can do tamasic work on the surface of the body. All you need is the right intention. From your reading of the aforegoing it might have seemed that I never do deep tamasic work, but the truth is I use it all the time. It is just that I do it from the surface and allow my energy to reach the appropriate depth, which is a relatively painless experience for the client. I trust the energy to do the work necessary to clear blockages. I decided a long time ago that to use negatively charged contacts and to feel that I had to go physically deep into the tissues simply meant that I really did not trust the life force, or that the quality of my intention had anything to do with the process. The release of energy blocks by using surface lever contacts and modulating the polarities, touches 1, 4, and 7, is, from my experience, a relatively painless process for the client apart from the occasionally intense sensations that occur as the blockage lets go. Detoxification happens at a natural rate that is easily supported by the client's eliminative capacity.

It is my opinion that there is nothing that can be achieved by the tamasic work as described by Dr. Stone that cannot be achieved by far more gentle methods. I suspect his work was enormously influenced by his original training in the physical techniques of chiropractic and osteopathy, some of which, as I know from personal experience, are quite ferocious. It is a tribute to his sensitivity and creativity that he was able to change his work from the physical to the energetic. I understand he also said that all students of Polarity Therapy should read and study his books and then move on from there. In this day and age when there are so many incredibly subtle energy-based techniques being developed, I cannot help but wonder about the personality of practitioners who use a lot of deep painful work on their clients. Is it just that they have a certain sadistic streak or a lot of blocked fire energy that they are trying to work through at their client's expense? Deep tamasic work can be very confrontational, and whilst there are perhaps occasions when confrontation is valid, as a general practice I do not see how it can be justified. Interestingly, you can get a lot of emotional release from deep tamasic work, but unfortunately it is not really the kind of spontaneous release that can be so important in a client's movement towards health. It is basically an emotional response to pain. We can all cry and be upset when we are feeling physical pain, but it is just a response, not the expression of a causative factor. I have heard it argued that it can help a person to release their fire energy, but the chances of a client with a fire problem being able to confront the powerful position the therapist occupies is not perhaps impossible but is highly unlikely.

If you have picked up the message during your Polarity training that emotional release is an important part of the therapeutic process you were taught well. However, if you think that deep tamasic work is a way of fulfilling this requirement then you are on the wrong track. What you need to do is refine your intention and your energetic sensitivity so that you are spontaneously drawn to the places in the client's energy field where the emotions are being held. All you need to do then is make a contact with the energy, create some movement and the emotions will come up. At that point remember the golden rule, Do Not Panic, just be there with them and allow it to change.

There are a few important points that you should bear in mind if you decide that you want to use the classic version of tamasic touch. Pressure applied to an area is a force acting at right angles to the contact surface. If you do not apply the force at right angles to the contact surface you will bring into play frictional forces. Working on someone's spine using a strong tamasic touch you should apply the force at right-angles to the surface of the skin. This is particularly important if you are working over the transverse processes of a vertebra. Should you apply the force at any other angle than at right angles to the flat surface of the transverse process you will create friction and shearing stresses in relation to the other bones. This is very painful for the client and is potentially dangerous, as should the forces become too great it is quite possible that you might damage the bone structure. These factors are even more critical if you use your elbow to do deep tissue work. However, this is not to say that you should never apply force at any other angle than right angles to the contact surface. You should be aware that when you do so the amount of pressure put on a particular area immediately increases because of the force vectors involved. The angled diagonal force you apply consists of two main components, the amount of pressure acting at an angle plus the additional frictional force that in effect prevents your hand from sliding off the contact area.

When doing any kind of rajasic work that involves rocking the body you should be aware that any body that is made to oscillate has a natural frequency. This frequency is determined by the body's mass in relation to the axis around which it is moving. As an example, a simple pendulum will swing quickly with a short length of string and the same pendulum will swing more slowly the longer the string gets. What this means in relation to a rajasic rocking movement that brings a client's whole body into oscillation is that it will be relatively of a much lower frequency than should you be rocking one leg from the hip. The natural frequency, for whichever section of the body you are rocking, is the rhythm that is maintained with the least amount of added force. This is easily felt because you will be able to maintain that rhythm with little effort. It is the same principle that applies when you are pushing a child on a swing. At a certain point you will be able to maintain their swinging movement with just a very small additional push every now and then. Part of the key to sensing the natural frequency is to maintain a high level of relaxation in your own shoulders and arms so that you can more clearly sense the responses in the clients body.

Rajasically stimulating the body as a whole or any particular part, at its natural frequency, nearly always gets the best energetic release possible. Just as in pushing a child on a swing, you do not follow the child as it swings continually pushing, you actually wait for the swing to come back to you before applying the next push. When rocking the body you do not follow the movement continually forcing the frequency, you allow the elasticity of the body to bring it back into your hand, having completed a cycle of movement before applying the next push. Should you apply the next push too soon or too late you will either change the frequency to one other than the natural one or you will stop the oscillation altogether. Working at the natural frequency is relatively effortless and this allows you to very easily sense any changes in the amount of force needed to maintain the oscillation. This is useful in that you can instantly sense any shifts in the tension patterns and energetic balance of a particular body area. It can occasionally be difficult to find the natural frequency, either because a client is actively trying to help the movement, or because sometimes the movement is masked by tension patterns in other areas of the body or you are holding too much tension in your own body. Generally speaking, after rocking for a short while any interference eases and you can then pick up the natural frequency.

One very general principle I use throughout my practice is that I never ask a client to do anything they could possible fail at. This principle applies throughout, even to something as simple as the response I give to a new client who, when getting on the table asks, "Is there anything I should do." My reply is always simply, "No, you can stay as tense as you like." When I say that the usual response is a wry smile or a chuckle, then they simply let go and relax.

The normal temptation may be to say that all they need to do is relax, in reply to this type of question. Yet, relaxation is, for most people, quite difficult. If you do give a client that kind of instruction, as they first lie on the table, you will inevitably get a lot of pointless wriggling around as they *try* and relax and ultimately fail. You might imagine an internal dialogue along the lines of, "Oh, No! I am terrible at relaxing, if this therapy relies on me being able to relax then its doomed to fail from the start." This kind of inner dialogue is profoundly unhelpful to the healing process.

It is really worth monitoring your own instructions to clients, in terms of things you would like them to do, either on the bodywork table or in relation to self-help, to see if you are actually instructing them to do things that they are going to routinely fail at.

2. Taking the Case History

Taking a client's case history is basically an in-depth information gathering process. The greater the clarity you have concerning the nature of a client's problems and their etiology, he more likely you are to be able to create effective therapeutic interventions. Taking the case history is definitely linked to your overall diagnosis. The basic skill necessary for taking an accurate case history is to be able to listen, but no less important is your visual perception. The skill of listening encompasses not just hearing what the client has to say, but knowing the right questions to ask that will elicit the most relevant information.

The most fundamentally important questions to ask when taking a case history are *what, how, where and when*. You are basically trying, in the first phase of information gathering, to define the actual nature of the client's problem. The very first question that I ask a client is 'How can I help you?' The questions that you ask after this first question are always aimed towards clarifying their answer. In fact, this is an ongoing process, each new question that you ask is always to clarify the preceding answer.

The usage of your visual skill comes into play whilst the client is answering your questions. Basically you are watching their body language as they answer. Are they tense, are they relaxed, how are they sitting, what kind of hand gestures are they making, are their legs or feet moving? Your visual field of perception needs to be wide enough to encompass their whole body. To do this you must not sit too close to the client, so give some forethought to the layout of your treatment room. The reason that the client's body language is so important is that it allows you to access information in relation to your questions that the client is not consciously aware of, because all body language is generated by the client's sub-conscious mind.

For example, suppose you ask a client about the quality of their intimate personal relationships and their reply to this is that they are fine and that they have no problems in this area, yet as they give this verbal response their body suddenly becomes tense or agitated; this could lead you to believe that in spite of what they said there was definitely some problem in this area, or, to use a Polarity term, that there was a 'charge' associated with this subject. We could say that you are experiencing an incongruity between the client's words and their body language. In fact, picking up on incongruent statements in relation to previous statements or body language is perhaps the most important aspect in obtaining a valid case history. It is important to remember that it is quite common for a client to lie to you without realizing that they are doing so because their own awareness of their problems is often limited. Any time you pick up an incongruity, at whatever level, always explore that area from another angle either there and then or at a later time. In your further questioning do not ever accuse the client of lying because what you are really dealing with is either sub-conscious suppression or self deception. We are all prone to manifesting these processes, which are fundamentally protective in nature.

Note Taking

Unless you have a truly phenomenal memory you are going to have to make notes as you take the case history, either in great detail or at least noting the most salient points. The ability to maintain an uninterrupted flow of conversation whilst at the same time taking notes is essential. Sometimes it is useful to create a standardized case history form that you can fill out for each new client. Such a form would have a space for the client's name, address, date of birth, presenting problem, medication, previous illnesses, previous treatment, diet, sleep patterns, leisure pursuits, occupation, marital status, children and so on. The actual areas that the form covers would be those areas that you feel are most important in relation to how you work. Such a form can also have a space for writing down the actual treatments that you give, and can become an important record for insurance purposes.

At the beginning in taking a case history most of the information exchanged revolves around what is called the 'presenting illness.' The presenting illness is quite often not the real problem that has to be dealt with but is only the surface level of imbalance. It is the problem area that is most familiar to the client but which is often only an effect not an actual cause. Very often the presenting illness will have a label or name given to it by the client's doctor, or sometimes by another alternative medical practitioner. If that is so make a note of it and then dismiss it from your consciousness. If it is a named disease that you are not familiar with then by all means look it up in a medical dictionary, but remember Polarity Therapy deals with energetic imbalances not physical diseases. What you really want to know is exactly how a particular named presenting illness affects them physically, mentally, emotionally.

If a client comes to you and says that they have arthritis of the knee, all that actually tells you is that a doctor has given them a label for their problem. It tells you nothing about how they experience the arthritis. Diseases are always individual, even though broadly speaking it may be possible to label them by defining certain features common to a wide range of symptoms. The kind of things you need to know when trying to ascertain a client's individual experience of a particular problem are: is it a constant experience or does the pain or awareness of the imbalance vary throughout the day? does it vary over a period of a week? what does any pain they experience actually feel like? is it hot, cold, sharp, dull, etc? Always try and get as much detail as possible concerning their particular problem.

Having looked at the presenting illness in depth it is important to then begin working back through all a client's past illnesses. You should look at the recent past of the last few years, but sometimes it is relevant to go as far back as their early childhood. What you are trying to do here is obtain a broad picture of all their past problems, how long they lasted, the kind of treatment they received and so forth. What you are looking for is a pattern of imbalances over the years. Sometimes you will also discover the causative factor of their current problems. I once had a client who came with abdominal distention and constipation which had been a problem for a number of years, which was, I suspect, initially triggered by having a difficult pregnancy some seven years previously. She had become anaemic, been given large doses of iron and became very constipated as a result. Her body, it seemed, had never properly recovered from the side effects of the treatment she received for the anaemia.

Once you have built up a picture of a client's current and previous state of health, you need to get some sense of the kind of life they lead. Are they married? do they have children? what sort of work do they do? what do they do in their spare time? what do they do to relax? are they satisfied with their life as a whole? what are the problem areas? All these questions and many others are useful in trying to come to some understanding of the kind of life a client leads. One area that can be very useful to explore is that of any major breaks in a client's life; by that I mean the death of relatives or other important people, change of occupation, moving house, divorce or separation, birth of children or a child leaving home. All these particular points in a person's life are extremely stressful and can have an enormous effect on their wellbeing. Do not be surprised if a client seems somewhat inarticulate when it comes to talking about themselves; it may be the first time anyone has actually asked them these kind of questions.

After getting a picture of the client's life style, the next important area is to find out what kind of diet they eat. The simplest way to do this is to ask them to go through a typical day's food consumption, describing what they eat at each meal. Apart from checking what they eat at main meal times, find out if they eat between meals. Ask them about their daily fluid intake, how much and what it is, and do not forget that such phrases as 'four cups of coffee a day' are relatively meaningless as the size of cups varies enormously. There is a great deal of difference between instant and espresso coffee. Make sure that you obtain precise answers. Do not forget to check alcohol intake. If you have not already done so this is a good point at which to check on what kind of drugs they take, not just prescription ones for particular problems but drugs like aspirin, paracetamol or 'recreational' drugs. An up-to-date dictionary of drugs is of invaluable help when trying to sort out what the possible effects and side effects of the drugs might be. Keep watching the client's body language!

The amount of time needed to take a case history can vary from fifteen minutes to around three-quarters of an hour. It really depends upon how articulate the client is about their particular problems. Sometimes, I have felt that I would have been more successful trying to get blood out of a stone than getting some basic case history information out of certain clients. It is important to remember that if a client has been 'trained' in the procedures of orthodox medicine, then the whole alternative holistic approach to health care can be quite a shock. Effectively your first job, apart from getting a full case history, is to educate them in holistic health care and preventative medicine.

It is important to realize that the process of taking a case history becomes an ongoing process as the client continues in therapy. At the beginning of each session a portion of time is always spent in review. One of the first questions that I ask at the beginning of each session is, "Tell me what has happened since I last saw you", or something similar. At this point you need to know what changes have occurred before you can proceed with treatment. Many of the questions that you asked in taking your first case history will still be relevant, and the answers you get will in all probability be different. The time needed to obtain the updated case history is nearly always much less than the original, perhaps only ten to fifteen minutes. Occasionally it can take much longer, particularly if the client feels happier and more confident about the nature of the work you are doing. It can be surprising what you learn during the second session.

Establishing Rapport

Ultimately, taking a good case history depends upon your ability to get a client to open up and express themselves freely. This is dependent upon the amount of rapport that you can establish with them. To create a good rapport between yourself and a client is to establish a relationship with them in which they can feel safe and secure. A feeling of security is vital to the free flow of what is often quite intimate and personal information. The process of creating a good rapport with a client depends on many factors but they can all be encapsulated in the concept of 'resonance.' Resonance is one of the most important concepts in Polarity Therapy. It comes into play in all areas of treatment, from taking the case history to the energy balancing bodywork.

When two vibrating objects whose fundamental or basic frequency is the same are brought together they will resonate. When two objects resonate the volume or amplitude of the particular frequency at which they vibrate will increase enormously. They are then said to form a resonating system. However, in the first instance should one of the objects not be vibrating, then as the other actively vibrating object is brought towards it will force or entrain a response in the inactive object, making it vibrate at the same frequency, and then they will be able to resonate together as a system. The classic example of this is the school physics experiment used to demonstrate the principle of resonance and entrainment, in which two tuning forks of the same frequency are used to represent the resonating system. Holding a tuning fork in each hand you tap one of the forks firmly against a hard surface to set it vibrating at its natural frequency, and then bring it slowly towards the other fork. At a certain distance apart the non-vibrating fork will suddenly begin to vibrate as the vibrating fork forces or entrains it to respond. They are then vibrating in harmony and are in resonance.

The principle of resonance applies to any vibrating objects. The human body and its energy field most definitely constitute a vibrating object, and any two or more people can constitute a resonating system. Indeed, because of the complexity of the human body, mind and energy system it can even be said to form a resonating system within itself. Much of the actual energy maps and balancing techniques are based upon this principle. If you understand the physics of music and the concept of harmonics you understand the basis of Polarity Therapy. When giving a Polarity treatment it is obvious that the practitioner and client constitute a resonating system. The client, because of their pain and illness, would be the inactive, non-vibrating part of the system; the therapist the active vibrating part who will entrain a similar response in the client, thereby effectively helping the client to return to full health. This concept gives us another definition of health in relation to human beings. To be healthy is to vibrate fully at your natural frequency.

This principle should not put you off giving a treatment when you are not feeling good, because in the human being it is predominantly the energy that is responsible for the resonance, and the state of your energy is ultimately controlled by your mind or consciousness. Giving a treatment is one of the best ways I know of becoming one-pointed in your consciousness and freeing your energy. The other point about a resonating system is that it is a reciprocal or two-way process. You could say that every time you give a Polarity treatment you receive a Polarity treatment.

The process of resonance begins with the first true contact that you have with the client, the first session. Taking the case history is really the first opportunity that you have to do anything of a practical nature towards the process of entrainment. As I mentioned earlier the term for this process during the case history taking is 'rapport.' To create a good rapport with a client involves the process of **pacing**, which itself has two main elements, *matching* and *mirroring*.

In essence, pacing is a technique for entering the client's reality. In practice this means that you should pay attention to the kind of language structure and content that the client uses, and modify your own to something similar. You are then matching their style of communication. This will ensure that the client has the best possible chance of understanding both your questions and any information of an educational nature that you might want to share with them. I touched on this concept in the previous chapter when discussing the kind of difficulties involved in explaining to a client exactly what Polarity Therapy is and how it works. However, matching does more than simply improve communication. It subtly creates a commonality of experience between you and the client, and this makes it very much easier for you to understand the nature of their problems. It is a mistake to believe that we all inhabit the same world. There are in fact something like four billion different ones in total, here on one quite small planet.

Mirroring is basically making your body posture and gestures a mirror of the client's own. This is a natural phenomena that occurs all the time in our everyday lives. Just watch two strangers on a park bench sometime and you will see that after a while they will mirror each other's positions. In the therapeutic environment such mimicry should be done subtly, otherwise if you make what you are doing too obvious the client will feel that you are making fun of them.

Another aspect to pacing is to allow yourself to become aware of the client's breathing rhythm and match your own to it. This particular form of matching is very powerful, as it is moving in to the realm of energetic matching which can create a profound change in the client's state of consciousness. The overall process of pacing is done by any good therapist more or less unconsciously, regardless of whether they have any understanding of the concept. Now that you have an understanding of the concept just watch yourself with a part of your awareness the next time you give someone a Polarity session to see when you are actually doing it. I can guarantee that you do it some of the time. Simply notice when you do it and have the thought that it will happen more often. Trying to force yourself to use pacing all the time tends to create a rather gross quality to what should be, and in normal everyday experience is, a subtle phenomena. Creating good rapport should be something that happens as easily as breathing and with as little attention. Allowing something to happen, once you have an understanding of it, is the best way to utilize new information. Very often 'trying' to do something seems to invoke the psychological equivalent of Newton's third law of motion that states 'for every action there is an equal and opposite reaction.'

One other tool that can be very useful in taking the case history is a five element check list. Basically this is a sheet of paper with the various elements and their functions listed

Five Element Check List:

ETHER		AIR		FIRE		WATER		EARTH	
JOINTS	☐	SHOULDERS	☐	EYES	☐	BREAST	☐	NECK	☐
		KIDNEYS	☐	SOLAR PLEXUS	☐	GENITALS	☐	BOWELS	☐
		ANKLES	☐	THIGHS	☐	FEET	☐	KNEES	☐
HEARING	☐	TOUCH	☐	VISION	☐	TASTE	☐	SMELL	☐
THROAT	☐	CHEST	☐	HEAD	☐	PELVIS	☐	ABDOMEN	☐
		CIRCULATION	☐	VITALITY	☐	SKIN	☐	BONES	☐
SPACY	☐	LOVING	☐	JOYFUL	☐	BALANCED	☐	STRONG	☐
GRIEF	☐	GREED	☐	ANGER	☐	LUSTFUL	☐	FEARFUL	☐

Fig. 1

in tabular form with small boxes, beside each category, for you to tick if the client has a disturbance in that particular area or function.

A sample checklist is reproduced in Fig. 1. It is by no means a definitive version and I suggest you create your own. I have found them very useful in creating a visual model of a client's imbalances. It allows you to see at a glance, when fully filled out, where the predominant disturbance is. In the sample chart you would tick the box if there was any kind of disturbance for that area but you could use other parameters of your own choosing to create a more specific representation.

3. Diagnosis

Diagnosis, like taking a case history, is an ongoing process that is important in every session that you give. To diagnose properly you need to re-evaluate the client's condition at the beginning of each session and also during actual treatment. It is possible to separate diagnosis into two categories, physical and energetic. Dr. Stone wrote extensively concerning physical diagnosis and so we will begin our look at the diagnostic process here. Some people prefer the term *assessment* rather than the more medical sounding term *diagnosis* but practically speaking there is no difference other than linguistically.

Physical Procedures

Physical diagnostic procedures are based upon the convenience of the patient, that is to say, they should all be done at the beginning of the session before the actual bodywork begins, and as far as possible should not involve the client having to get on and off the table a number of times unless you are doing a structural session. The first diagnostic procedure is done using the gravity board to ascertain the way in which the client organizes their physical structure in relation to gravity. This subject is dealt with in depth in the chapter on structural balancing later in this book. The second diagnostic procedure is taking the client's blood pressure. This is most conveniently done with the client sitting on the bodywork table. It should be taken on both sides of the body because the information so gained can be very useful in relation to balancing of the autonomic nervous system using perineal and coccygeal treatments. Remember that even though a client's blood pressure may register high, this is no reason to suppose that it is so at other times. There are many factors that can influence the blood pressure at the beginning of a treatment, not the least being nervous anticipation. The pulse rate may also be taken at this time. The radial pulse should be taken at both sides, as should the pulse at the carotid artery. Currently, there are available automated digital devices that register both blood pressure and pulse simultaneously, some even work by checking the blood pressure at the fingers which is infinitely more useful in that the blood pressure and pulse rate can be monitored throughout the session. When checking the pulse rate manually, do it quickly with a light touch as it is quite easy to create a false reading because excessive finger pressure influences it very quickly. The pulse can also be taken at other places on the body, which allows you to build up a picture of the overall distribution of life energy to the various areas of the body.

The third procedure is done with the client lying on the bodywork table, and it is to ascertain the short leg side. The short leg side indicates the side of the body on which there is an overall contraction of the electromagnetic currents of energy. It is basically caused by unequal muscle tension in the pelvis, and is a partial indicator of sacral positioning. It can be caused by physical injury or by a functional imbalance in the five elements. See p. 218 for more on measuring the short leg side

The fourth procedure is to check the respiratory functioning. This is most easily done by placing your hands in different positions on the client's rib cage and checking the mobility of the different areas, as the client breathes both normally and when encouraged to breathe deeply. After doing this, check the respiratory rate, the number of breaths that they take per minute. This gives you the overall picture of the functioning of the sympathetic nervous system. It tells you how much oxygen and prana the client is drawing from the atmosphere. You can correlate the number of breaths per minute to the pulse rate. A good balance is four heartbeats to every one breath. Should the respiratory rate be very slow and the pulse fast, then you could interpret this as indicating that whilst the circulation of energy may be good the actual quantity may be far less than is necessary for adequate functioning of the body.

Dr. Stone liked to check the nasal passages to see whether they were sufficiently open to allow a free flow of breath and prana. He also recommended using gold and silver dilators to open the passages. This is a technique that was developed at the turn of the century and works on the sympathetic reflex areas in the Shneiderian membrane of the nasal cavity. However, this technique is far beyond the scope of this book. You can effect a dilation of the nasal passages by doing deep breathing exercises using the alternate nostril breathing techniques of the yogic science of pranayama or more modern approaches such as the Buteyko method. It is important to encourage nasal breathing as it has a number of distinct advantages over mouth breathing. As the air passes through the nostrils it is cleaned and filtered by the hairs in the nose as well as being heated to a level that will not harm the sensitive internal membranes of the throat and lungs. The prana in the breath is absorbed directly into the brain via the nasal membranes and sinuses where it activates the cerebral cortex and the caduceus currents of energy.

The next thing to look at is exactly how the client's body is lying on the table. Look for any kind of angular distortions in the way that it is lying. For example you may find that the head and the torso seem balanced and symmetrically aligned, but that from the diaphragm area the body seems to veer off to the right or left (Fig. 2). It is possible that

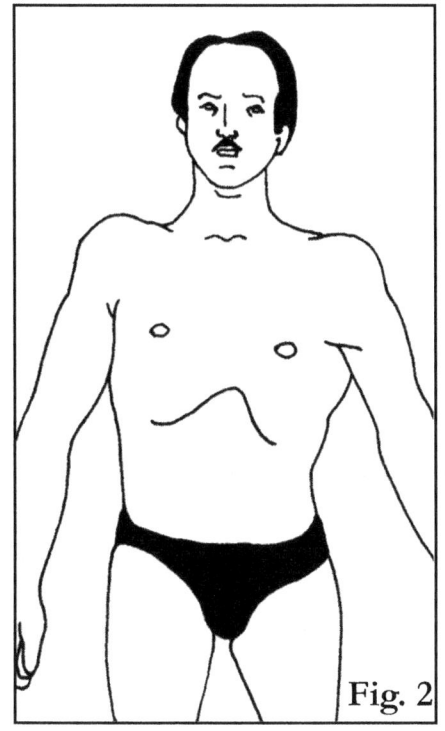

Fig. 2

a client may show a number of angular distortions so that they are lying in a zigzag fashion on the table. These angular distortions nearly always occur at the different chakra levels and are indicative of disturbances at the point where the distortion occurs (see Fig. 77 and Fig. 78 p. 170). These distortions are indicative of imbalances in the flow of life energy in the body. They are not gravity related structural distortions because as the body is lying on the table gravity is no longer acting on it to the extent that it does when standing. What you see as the client is lying on the table is the way the mind, emotions and the flow of life energy directly affect the muscle structure and bodily alignment. When off gravity the position that the physical body adopts is a direct reflection of the inner flow of life energy without any primary adaptation to gravity. This is because, as Dr. Stone pointed out, the life energy and the five elements are beyond the influence of gravity. Ideally this kind of body and energy reading would best be done with the client suspended in water. Unfortunately, this is not practical in the average treatment room! When reading the body in this way always look from the top of the table down the client's body and from the bottom of the table up, as it is sometimes easier to see distortions from one angle rather than another. What you are seeing is, in a sense, the client's inner relationships, how they feel about themselves, the dynamics of their self image and character structure. I shall explore this topic in much greater detail in the chapter on structural balancing. Unlike some therapies where it is recommended that the client is positioned symmetrically on the table, to do so in a Polarity session is to lose out on the opportunity to gather a great deal more information towards your overall diagnosis.

It is also useful to check for hot and cold areas on the client's body. This is done by using the hands to pick up actual differences in the surface temperature. You are using your hands to detect problems with circulation, which is indicated predominantly by warm and cool areas. The hot areas are indicative of inflammation and excessive energy. Very cold areas are indicative of chronic energy blocks. Whilst this technique is quite useful, you have to be able to make some kind of differentiation between the terms warm, cool, hot and cold in relation to each client individually. It is important that the room is uniformly heated and that the client has been undressed and lying still for some five to ten minutes before trying to use this kind of diagnosis.

The final aspect of physical diagnosis is looking at the alignment and possible disfigurement of the fingers and toes. The finger and toe nails are reliable indicators of energetic disturbances, in as much as dryness, brittleness, splitting, discolouration, ridging of any particular finger or toe can be related to some kind of disturbance in the element, chakra and organs represented by it. As disturbances of the feet are indicative of chronic conditions and the hands of acute conditions, any severe disfiguration in the finger nails shows a chronic or dormant condition that is now becoming active. Usually such a disturbance in the finger nail will be matched by a similar problem with the related toe nail. The alignment of the fingers and toes is another useful diagnostic indicator, in that twists, bends and overlapping are also indicative of problems in the related areas of the body. A lack of mobility in any of the joints is another important factor.

Another useful diagnostic indicator is the amount of retained circulation in the fingertips when they are squeezed. The amount of retained circulation indicates the degree of energy flowing in any of the corresponding areas represented by that finger. To do this one simply squeezes the sides of the tip of the finger to see the amount of circulation retained under the nail. It is also useful to study the rate at which the blood returns when the finger is released. Check all the fingers and compare. Remember that the blood carries the bulk of prana in circulation in the body, so all the diagnosis based on blood flow is a direct indicator of energy flow. You can also sense differences in the circulation by squeezing the fingertips quickly and gently and comparing the elasticity and fullness of the tissue.

Pulse Diagnosis

The bridge between purely physical diagnosis and purely energetic is the art of Ayurvedic pulse diagnosis. The blood is, as I said, the main carrier of the life energy. It is made up of three principles: the airy principle, which relates physically to the oxygen within the blood and energetically is the prana; the fire principle, which is the heat within the blood stream; and the water principle, which is the basic fluidic nature of blood. The pulse beat depends on these three principles for its rhythm and quality. In Ayurvedic pulse diagnosis the pulse is taken with the tips of the air, fire and water fingers. The information obtained relates physically to the pumping of the heart, the elasticity of the arteries and capillary pressure, and energetically to the three principles or, to use the Ayurvedic term, the three Doshas. The Doshas, which should not be confused with the five elements although they are related, are Vayu (air), Pitha (fire) and Kapha (water). The Doshas are the Ayurvedic term for the three forces that are active in any disease state or physical disharmony. They are perhaps most easily understood by the terms 'dry problems,' 'hot problems,' and 'watery problems,' so any physical problem can be characterized by being caused by either too much or too little air, heat or water within the body. In Polarity terms the three Doshas could perhaps be understood as being related to the terms positive, neutral and negative. In which case, the air dosha would be the neutral phase of movement of energy, the fire dosha would be related to the positive phase of energy movement, and the water dosha to the negative phase. The Doshas are related to the five elements in the following way: the air dosha is a combination of the ether and air elements; the fire dosha is either the fire element alone or sometimes in combination with the water element (different schools of Ayurvedic medicine disagree on this); and the water dosha is a combination of the water and earth elements.

Qualities of the Doshas

VAYU (Air)

is the moving force of the living body and without it the other two doshas could not move. It is concerned with physical and mental processes which are dynamic in nature; sight, speech, hearing, etc., and perceptions in all physical and psychic manifestations. It sets and keeps in motion all other forces which are incapable of moving on their own. Vayu governs enthusiasm, respiration, motor activities (mental and physical). It regulates the autonomic nervous system. It manifests itself in any inflammatory state as pain. No pain is possible without Vayu. Vayu is light, cold, dry, mobile and piercing.

PITHA (Fire)

is to heat, to bum or warm up. It is concerned with physical and mental processes which are balancing and transformative in nature; hunger, cheerfulness, intelligence, ideas, digestion, thirst. The function of Pitha is to regulate and maintain oxidation and supply heat as well as maintain thermal balance within the body.

KAPHA (Water)

is the equivalent of cold in the body. It embraces and holds things together. It modifies and checks Pitha. It lubricates the body, especially the joints and skin. Kapha supports tissue growth. It produces courage, forbearance and vitality. Kapha is conserving and stabilizing in its effect.

As you can see, there is a definite relationship between the doshas and the elements, and from my own personal study of Ayurvedic medicine it seems to me that the three principles or doshas were conceptualized because Ayurvedic doctors found that the five element theory was too complicated when trying to devise appropriate therapeutic strategies.

To take the pulse you use the air, fire and water fingers of your right hand. When taking the pulse of a male client you take it at his right wrist, and of a lady client at her left wrist. The client's pulse is taken in such a way that your air finger is always the finger nearest to the base of the thumb. Its exact position is two finger-widths below the root of the thumb. The pulse is taken with the client sitting down. The client's arm is bent slantingly upwards, supported at the elbow by your free hand (Fig. 3). Their hand should be held so that the fingers point upwards as you take the pulse.

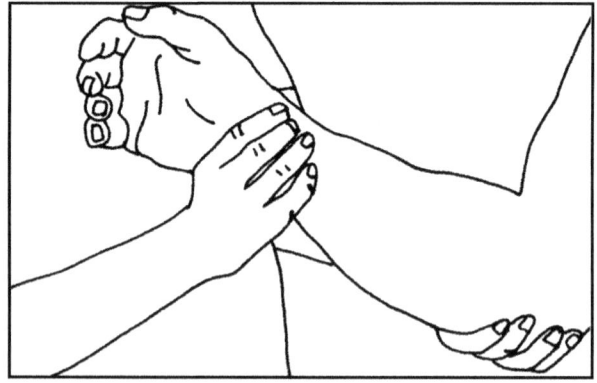

Fig. 3

Do not try to take a client's pulse if they have just had a bath, shower, or meal, or if they have been exercising. Nor should they be hungry or thirsty. Basically, they need to be calm both mentally and physically.

Once you can feel the pulse you need to get a sense of what is happening under all three of your fingers. You are sensing the activity over quite a long section of the radial pulse.

In Ayurvedic medicine there are considered to be some six hundred different pulse qualities. We are just going to look at a few of the main variations. The pulsation that you feel under the air finger relates to Vayu, under the fire finger relates to Pitha and under the water finger relates to Kapha. Firstly, it is always a good idea to define what that rarest of animals—a normal pulse beat—feels like. It is a pulse that can be felt under all three fingers with the sensation under each finger being slow, light and forceful. You should also be able to exert moderate pressure on the pulse without it being obliterated. It can only exist when all the three doshas are in harmony. Looking at the doshas individually the pulses related to them are:

> *Vayu* a fast pulse, which feels as if it moves in curves like a snake.

> *Pitha* a jumpy pulse. Its movement is like that of a frog or sparrow.

> *Kapha* a slow pulse. Its movement is like that of a swan or peacock.

When sensing the pulse through your fingertips the first thing to ascertain is where you feel it. If it impinges mainly on your air finger then Vayu is out of balance, on your fire finger then Pitha is out of balance or on your water finger then Kapha is out of balance. If the pulse feels as though it is between the air and fire fingers, then both Vayu and Pitha are disturbed, and between your fire and water fingers then Pitha and Kapha are disturbed. If the pulse seems to come between all three fingers then all the doshas are out of balance. If you feel the pulse at all three fingertips but more strongly at one than the others, then the dosha corresponding to the finger where the pulse is strongest is disturbed. Having decided where you are feeling the pulse look to its quality. Is it fast, slow, or jumpy? Or to use the animal symbology, is it moving like a snake, a swan or a frog? If it at first seems fast and snakelike, then becomes jumpy or froglike and finally moves slowly like a swan, then the doshas are functioning in a regular fashion and this indicates an excellent prognosis in terms of the client making a full recovery. When all three doshas are disturbed the pulse will seem to be fast, slow and jumpy all at once. When the pulse moves alternately like a snake and then a frog, both Vayu and Pitha are disturbed. If it moves like a snake and then a swan, Vayu and Kapha are disturbed, and should it move like a frog and then a swan both Pitha and Kapha are in trouble.

The technique as outlined above is, I hope, clear and simple enough for anyone to learn the fundamentals of Ayurvedic pulse diagnosis. The only way to become skilful is through constant practice. Learning any of the oriental techniques of pulse diagnosis is a lifelong process, but the usefulness of the skill more than justifies the effort.

The other form of diagnosis which I also see as a bridge between the physical and the purely energetic procedures is foot and hand reflexology. I do not propose to go into these techniques in detail as they have been dealt with in great depth in the many excellent books available on the subject. However, a couple of points seem worth mentioning. Occasionally there are so many sore areas on a client's foot as to make you think that all their energy flows and related organs are disturbed. This phenomena is, in my experience, usually caused by a severe water element imbalance, very often in the pelvis. In this situation the hands will normally give a clearer picture. When checking the reflexes always flex the feet, as this helps to bring the reflexes to the surface.

Energetic Procedures

Energetic diagnosis, sometimes called clairvoyant or psychic diagnosis, is the direct sensing of the state of a client's energy field by hearing, touch or vision. There is no 'sixth sense' involved in this process. It is done by developing an acute degree of sensitivity in one or more of the aforementioned senses. The most commonly developed channels for the information to be obtained through are sight and touch, though it is possible to 'hear' the energy, particularly by people with highly developed musical 'ear.' Energy is, after all, vibration just as is sound. My own particular skills are in sensing energy by touch and vision, so techniques that use these two senses are the ones I shall look at in detail.

Using a Pendulum

Before looking at these techniques it is important to note that there is another technique that can be used to diagnose a client's condition, and this is by the use of a pendulum. A pendulum is simply a small, heavy weight made of either wood, metal or crystal that is attached to a piece of string or a chain that is about six to eight inches (fifteen to twenty cm) long. Pendulum diagnosis can be done even before you see a client, which is worth doing from the point of view of not making the client think that you are a bit strange, and also as a way of checking the accuracy of your 'dowsing' (to use the correct term). After using a pendulum for a period of time and becoming proficient in its usage, you often find that you no longer need it because you know where the problems are immediately at a conscious level. Dowsing is a way of accessing your own sub-conscious mind. It is also a way of familiarizing yourself with the fact that you have a sub-conscious mind, an aspect of your consciousness which is intimately aware of life energy as it is the medium through which it controls the functioning of the body. It is through our sub-conscious mind and the fact that it can easily access information from the sub-conscious mind of the client, perhaps through the existence of the collective unconscious as well as some properties that are inherent in life energy, that we are able to diagnose the state of their energy. Using the pendulum is a way of training your sub-conscious mind in the particular language of energy that is used in Polarity Therapy until it can present it directly to your conscious awareness.

Learning to use the pendulum is very easy. All you need to do is calibrate it and then decide on the kind of questions you want to ask. To calibrate a pendulum is to clarify the kind of movement that it makes to indicate a 'yes' answer, and the movement that indicates a 'no' answer. When using the pendulum I have found it best if you support the elbow. Set the pendulum swinging very gently in a backwards and forwards oscillation (towards you and away from you) with a range of about one to two inches (three to five cm). Now ask the question either out loud or in your mind 'is my name ...' using your full name. This is a question which must get an affirmative response, so the way in which the pendulum moves in relation to this question is its 'yes' answer, which may be the same back and forth movement you began with or a different one. Once again set the pendulum swinging very gently. Now ask a question the answer to which you know is going to be 'no,' for example 'am I ... years old' using a figure that is definitely wrong. The direction of movement you get in response to this question is your 'no' answer. Commonly people find that a 'yes' answer is some kind of circular swing and a 'no' answer a side to side or back and forth movement, or sometimes 'yes' is a clockwise circle and 'no' an anticlockwise circle. There really are no set rules. Initially, it is best to check the calibration of the pendulum each time you use it until a set pattern is established. This usually only takes a short while but for the sake of accuracy it is worth doing at first.

The questions you ask in relation to a client's energy are almost limitless. You can ask about the functioning of the five elements, the activity of the chakras, the nervous system balance, check for blockages in the individual current lines, and so on. Always make sure that you understand the subject area that you are dowsing. In other words, if you do not understand the five element theory then do not ask questions about the balance of the elements, as the answers from the pendulum are not likely to be accurate. Remember it only reflects the understanding that your sub-conscious mind has of the language you are using, and if you do not understand elemental theory because you have not studied and comprehended it, how can you expect your sub-conscious to give you meaningful accurate answers. It is worth noting that using a pendulum in the manner I have outlined above is by no means the only way it can be used, any good book on dowsing will offer you many other possibilities.

Hand Scanning

What is often referred to as hand scanning is one of the simplest ways of feeling imbalances in the client's energy field. Remember that the energy field or aura extends way beyond the boundaries of the physical body. The aura itself is composed of many interpenetrating layers of energy, all vibrating at different frequencies. The layer of the aura that we are often most interested in is the so-called 'health aura,' or sometimes the etheric double, which is the particular vibrations of energy that radiate from the core of the energy field to no more than one-half to one inch beyond the surface of the body. To scan this layer of the aura simply run your open palm slowly all over the surface of the body approximately one inch above it. What you are looking for are changes in sensation in the palm of your hand. There is no specific quality of sensation that you should experience. What you want to feel are the differences between the various areas you are scanning. The kind of sensations that you might experience are predominantly a mixture of heat, cold, tingling, vibration, pain, pulsation or pressure. The actual sensation that you get when sensing energy is going to be unique to you. This is not a skill that comes quickly, but it certainly is one that is worth cultivating. Feeling disturbances in a client's energy field is only the first step of this particular kind of psychic diagnosis. The ability to interpret the sensations that you experience, what they actually mean, is something that could take you many years of practice to achieve with any degree of clarity. There are many books that purport to define the meanings of the various sensations that you can experience whilst hand scanning. However, because everyone's experience is subtly different, there is really no reason to suppose that the information contained in books of this kind is going to be useful to you.

It is important when hand scanning to move your hands slowly over the body, because the sensations that you experience are very subtle. If you move your hand too quickly you will not give yourself time to absorb the various impressions. It is almost as if there is a time lag between your sense of touch picking up some variation and your conscious recognition of it. Having said that you should do the technique slowly, if you do it too slowly you will actually begin to manipulate the flow of energy in that particular area just as if you were giving a treatment. If there is a rule when practicing hand scanning it is 'first impressions count.' Re-checking any particular area more than once will also affect the energy there. You can practice this technique on yourself, which can be particularly useful in learning to interpret what you are feeling, especially if you have some specific problem areas that are easy for you to reach and scan with your palm. Some people find that one of their hands is more sensitive than the other when doing this kind of diagnosis.

Quite often it is the left hand, but again it is a personal preference. Scanning the physical or health aura tells you a great deal about the physiological functioning of the body. It is also possible to scan the aura further from the body than the boundaries of the health aura, out into the layers of the aura that correlate with the different levels of the mind.

Scanning the auric shell between one to ten inches (three to twenty-five cm) off the body corresponds to the sub-conscious mind and emotions. It is sometimes called the astral area of the aura. Scanning from ten inches to two feet (twenty five to sixty cm) off the body corresponds to the conscious mind and thoughts, and from two feet (sixty cm) off the body to the boundaries of the aura (which varies) relates to the super-conscious mind and soul. Checking all of the aura from the physical to the super-conscious area can reveal much concerning an energy disturbance that you detect at the physical level, as should there be a disturbance further off the body in the same area you can deduce whether the problem has emotional, mental or spiritual factors involved. As some clients can find it rather strange if you scan the outer layers of the aura, not being used to seeing someone floating their hands some way off their body, I usually ask them to relax and close their eyes for a few moments whilst I do it. I personally find it something of a distraction watching the bemused expression on their face if they keep their eyes open!

What I call *deep scanning* is a variation of hand scanning. It involves projecting the energy from your palm down into the body to ascertain exactly where the source of the energy imbalance that is manifesting at the surface of the body actually is. The ability to detect the actual source of any particular energy disturbance can make your release work much more specific and effective. If you remember that all the different frequencies of life energy begin at the core and radiate outward, it is obvious that many of the disturbances that you detect in the physical aura will have their roots much deeper in the body's energy fields. The Hermetic concept of 'as within, so without' also relates to this phenomena. The actual technique is to place your hand on the surface of the body and project your energy like a beam which will be reflected back to you, the source, when it meets an obstacle. A radar or sonar beam acts in just this fashion when it meets an object. The effectiveness of this technique depends upon your awareness. Remember that your intention moves your energy. What you are looking for is an awareness of a resistance or a complete blockage to the free movement of your energy as you project it into the body. With practice it is possible to determine quite precisely the exact depth and size of any energy blockage in the client's energy field. Not all disturbances in the physical aura will be coming from a deeper level. When you place your hand on the body to do deep scanning and you have a feeling that your energy and awareness cannot penetrate beneath the surface, that they are scattered instantly, then you could expect that you were picking up tension or armouring in the superficial muscles in that area. When you come to trying to release the blockage that you have discovered, by whatever technique that you think appropriate, the perception that you have of its actual depth and position will enormously enhance the clarity of your intention, which in turn will ensure a full clearance of the energy field.

By working with energetic diagnostic techniques for some length of time and having become very familiar with the life energy after giving many sessions, you will probably find that you will begin to 'see' the energy. A visual as opposed to kinaesthetic perception of the life energy is not necessarily more accurate, but it is certainly faster. It is true to say that some people are far more adept at feeling the aura than they ever could be at seeing it. Indeed, I would say that everybody can learn to feel energy but not everyone can learn to see it. To be able to see something which is not physical requires the ability to let go of your normal everyday visual models of reality. For some people this is impossible, because it would mean a loss of psychological stability. Initially you will see the energy with your peripheral vision, out of the corner of your eye, so to speak. Do not try to chase or force the phenomena, just notice it when it happens and accept that it will probably become more frequent. There are various systems of eye exercises that are designed to facilitate your visual perception of the aura, and certainly they work for some people. To be able to see it really clearly requires you to be able to enter what is basically an altered state of consciousness, so meditation practice and experience with hypnotic states can be beneficial in helping to expand your world view to encompass the ability to see the energy that is the essence of life.

Ultimately, by continuing to practice all these diagnostic assessment techniques you will, in all probability, reach a point where your sub-conscious mind has assimilated them so well that you will simply 'know' what the sources of a client's energy imbalances are without actually performing any of the procedures outlined above. At this point you will have transcended technique and have moved into artistry.

4. Second Thoughts

The practice of Polarity Therapy lies in a grey area between Body-Orientated Psychotherapy and Alternative Medicine, the particular emphasis, be it psychotherapy or alternative medicine, being at the discretion of the individual practitioner. I believe that Polarity Therapy as taught and practiced by Dr. Stone was a powerful form of drugless healing, and so would come under the generic title of Alternative Medicine. The psychotherapeutic approach is a more recent development created by students who already had a background either in counseling or in the various body-orientated forms of psychotherapy such as Reichian Therapy or Bioenergetics. It will therefore be of some interest to look at the major current models of psychotherapeutic practice so as to see perhaps where your own approach lies.

Having a clear sense of the model that you are using with any particular client will give a better foundation upon which both you and your client can judge the effectiveness of the work and allow the contract between you to be unambiguous. It is also important to remember that you do have to limit yourself to using just one model in your practice. I have often found myself working for a few months as an alternative medical practitioner, followed by a few months as a psychotherapist and so on. Indeed, the model that you use often seems to be dictated by the universal law of attraction. If you are going through a period of emotional readjustment then those are the kind of clients you will attract and you will be doing psychotherapy, or if you are experiencing aches and pains or have recently injured yourself you will attract clients who need drugless healing. It all depends on exactly where your consciousness is at any particular time.

Content and Process Models

All current systems of psychotherapy have a therapeutic model, that is an overall concept of the way the particular system being used functions. Currently, the two major models in usage are content and process based therapy. These approaches can then be either strategic or client centred. The content model of psychotherapy is based upon the concept that for a resolution of the client's problems it is necessary for them to become consciously aware of the roots, at the sub-conscious level, of the reasons for their particular problem; in essence the belief being that if we know why we are doing or experiencing something that is a problem, it will change. It could also be called an insight model, in that it relies on insight into the nature and causes of a particular problem to provide a stimulus to change. The main content question is 'why?' The major problem with doing purely content-based therapy in this day and age is that people are fundamentally far more sophisticated in their understanding of psychological patterns, and unless the roots of their problems lie in an area with which they have no familiarity the insight gained will not have any appreciable impact on their problem. Freudian Psychoanalysis is the classic example of a therapy that uses a content model. In the time period in which it was developed, showing clients that the roots of their problems lay in the oedipal situation had an enormous psychological impact simply because it was not an area of human relationships that anyone had really previously looked at in any depth. I believe that there is in all of us a desire to know why something is the way it is. It is the basic drive behind all scientific discovery in every field, the essential curiosity of the human being without which we would still be living in caves. It is clear in Dr. Stone's writings that he believed in the insight model.

The process model is based upon the concept that it is not why we do something, but the process or the steps that cause a particular problem that are significant. An understanding of how we go about creating a particular problem is the main aim of process-orientated therapy. Once we understand how we create a particular problem we can then interfere consciously in the process or steps we would normally take and create a new outcome for ourselves. Process therapy focuses a great deal of attention on the flow of feelings in the mind-body continuum. It looks at such things as body movement, posture, voice tone, etc., as indicative of the feeling stream in relation to the content of any particular experience. Awareness practices often form a large part of process-orientated therapy, learning to become aware of tension patterns in the body, discovering how you feel about your body, and so on. Process questions are 'how, when, where, what?.' Gestalt therapy and Neuro- Linguistic Programming are examples of therapeutic systems that largely use the process model.

Strategic and Client Centred Approaches

Apart from the therapeutic model there is what I call the therapeutic approach. It is the basic structure of the relationship between therapist and client. There are two main approaches at this time, 'strategic' and 'client centred.' The strategic approach to therapy, be it based on the content or process model, occurs when the therapeutic techniques are decided by the therapist without consultation with the client. In the strategic approach the therapist's role is that of strategist who plans a campaign of action down to the finest details, who evaluates the effects of the actions taken, modifies any plans according to the responses and evaluates the outcome himself. Although the client will usually specify some kind of desired outcome during the initial consultation, if they do not the therapist will create a series of therapeutic changes based on his own evaluation of the client's needs. The strategic approach may well take a client far beyond any original request for a particular outcome. This sometimes happens because the strategy used to effect a particular outcome may have far greater ramifications than implied in the original request, and the techniques used create change at such a fundamental level that much more is derived from the therapy than the client originally intended. In the strategic approach the therapist takes full responsibility for the influence he exerts on the client. Ericksonian hypnotherapy is an example of strategic therapy.

The client-centred model is based upon the therapist initiating no therapeutic interventions until the client is able to articulate their needs. The idea being that if a client has a problem but does not know what to do about it, then the therapist should involve them fully in the decision making process by reflecting back their comments in a passive way until sufficient clarity develops in the mind of the client as to what they actually want out of the therapy. This is an ongoing element in the therapy, the client specifying the therapeutic outcome and being fully involved in the therapy, making new choices in full consultation with the therapist as the work progresses. There is an avoidance of any sense of manipulation of the client by the therapist as being 'dis-empowering,' as taking away their sense of being in control of their lives. In the client-centred approach the responsibility for the nature of the work lies with the client. Rogerian Therapy is the classic client centred approach and Humanistic psychology also tends to use the client-centred model.

To a great extent any but the most ardent purists within any particular system of psychotherapy will probably use more than one model in their practice. Nearly all practitioners of process-orientated therapy will make some content based interpretations at various points in their work. Practitioners of content-orientated therapy will also focus on process periodically. However, it would be rare to find a therapist who uses both the client-centred approach and the strategic approach. Most practitioners will opt for one of the approaches and stay with that throughout their working life as a therapist.

Most systems of psychotherapy have a particular conceptual model of the *healthy human being*. The definitions of such a person range from someone who is free of all neurosis, to a person capable of a full orgasm, to someone who is self-actualising. Any therapy is to a great extent orientated, whatever its model, to turning the client into its own vision of a healthy person. The existence of such models of a perfect human being means that whatever the desired outcome of the therapy as specified by the client, the course of the therapy must be subordinated to the therapist actualising within the client the model of perfect human functioning that they ascribe to. For instance, a client comes to a therapist whose model of perfect functioning is a person capable of a full orgasm. The client's specific desire is to overcome certain anxieties in relation to their working life, perhaps their ability to deal with authority figures. The only way that the therapist can achieve this is by seeking to make the client able to express their concept of perfect functioning, because if they can achieve this then all the client's problems will disappear. Admittedly, this is a simplistic interpretation of what is in fact an exceedingly complex process, but in essence it is a valid statement. It is as well to know the kind of concept of a healthy human being that a therapist subscribes to before undergoing any therapeutic work with them. These models often contain a number of inbuilt limitations that you may not wish to take on board.

As a Polarity therapist, what do you feel is your concept of a healthy human being? What was the model expressed during your training? In some training courses the model is not taught openly but has to be inferred from many different statements concerning human behavioural patterns. It is always possible to reduce the model offered, whether openly or covertly, no matter how seemingly complicated, to a few simple statements or even a single phrase. The Polarity concept of a healthy individual according to Dr. Stone is a person with abundant free flowing energy and who has a sense of connection with the source of all life, and to this I would add, who also has the ability to change easily.

The therapeutic contract, like any contract, is an agreement between two parties concerning some form of business arrangement. If you practice Polarity Therapy as a system of alternative medicine then the contract that you enter into with the client will be fairly simple. It will be to the effect that you as a therapist undertake to restore, as far as is possible, normal functioning in their body as quickly as is feasible, and that they undertake to come for a specified number of sessions or until the problem is resolved, and further that they will pay for this service. The important factor here is that it would be unwise, from the practitioner's point of view, to make any categoric statement to the effect that the client will definitely get better. It is as well to remember that in many countries it is against the law to make claims of possessing an ability to cure certain diseases. Any false or exaggerated claim on the part of the practitioner is going to undermine the relevance of any contract, if not totally invalidating it.

If you practice Polarity Therapy as a form of body and energy based psychotherapy then the contract between you and your client needs to cover a broader spectrum of issues. The practitioner's side of the contract needs to cover such details as cost; the number of sessions; the point at which some form of mutual review of therapeutic progress is undertaken; the kind of therapy that is offered; an explanation of the possible effects of the therapy and the confidentiality of personal information. It should also specify any ground rules to be followed during the actual session; for example, if you are doing a lot of counseling, is the client allowed to smoke? If you use some form of cathartic emotional release work, is violence against you prohibited or would it be permissible for the client to physically wrestle with you? Do you offer telephone support to the client outside of normal business hours? The client's side of the contract covers such issues as payment on time, punctuality, an agreement to offer, as far as is possible, information both honestly and openly, and that if any issues arise over which they are in any way unsure, they will clarify them with the practitioner. Actually going for therapy implies, at least at some level, a willingness on behalf of the client to change, which, if you like, is part of the implicit unspoken aspects of the contract.

My own opinion of the fundamental model on which Polarity Therapy is based is that it is a process model. Working with the life energy is working with the essential ground of being, the dance of life. It is impossible to talk about the flow of life energy in the body in terms of 'why.' The energy just 'is.' I use a strategic approach in the Polarity work that I do. I practice Polarity both as alternative medicine and psychotherapy. With some clients I find the work shifts from alternative medicine to psychotherapy during treatment, thereby necessitating the negotiation of a new contract.

There is the possibility of another model of approach to Polarity Therapy which is not client-centred or strategic, in that it does not offer the client any specific outcomes. It is non-directive and is not even 'therapy' in the normal usage of the term, although the effects can certainly be therapeutic. I call this approach the 'attunement approach.' It seeks to attune the client to the existence of life energy and its flow in the body through the experience of the energy work. It is all about giving the client an experience in its purest form without any interpretation or explanations. It is Polarity for personal growth in the sense of a growth in consciousness or knowingness of life, to know what it is to be 'alive.' It is trusting that the life energy has consciousness and wisdom, and that it will create the most appropriate changes in the client because the prana, the breath of life, is also the breath of the soul, and it is the soul that truly knows what we need and how we should be in this life. An attunement to the life energy is, when done properly, the creation of a channel of communication with a person's own soul. To practice Polarity Therapy in this way is to no longer be locked in a therapist/client relationship but to be joint adventurers in the exploration of the subtle realms.

The attunement approach involves a joining and resonance at the level of the soul, where two unique individuals, freed from the confines of matter, can soar and dance in the quest for the source of all life. It is the Taoist return to the source that is beyond death whilst still being fully involved in the process of life. This particular approach to Polarity is best attempted upon a solid foundation of practical and theoretical knowledge of the system. It is not an excuse for ineptitude. The attunement approach is an approach that transcends any concept of therapy, and could perhaps be expressed in the form of a Taoist paradox stated as 'Therapy, Non-Therapy,' or that one learns and practices therapy so that you do not have to do it. It is an approach that holds to the idea that the most effective therapeutic changes come out of a profound relationship between the people involved.

5. The Five Elements

One of the most fundamental aspects of Polarity Therapy is an understanding of the five element theory. Having studied Dr. Stone's books and many books on Ayurvedic medicine, as well as consulting with various people who were supposed to understand the theory, I found myself getting more and more confused. The main source of my confusion was a statement in Dr. Stone's writings to the effect that the five elements were like the plates in a battery which were energized by the life energy or prana. This seemed to indicate that he saw the five elements as energized substances, and yet I have also seen the theory stated that the five elements are fundamentally just five different qualities of energy in movement. Dr. Stone also wrote at various times of the five elements as matter and at other times as energy. My confusion only began to clear when I realized that in Ayurvedic medicine there are the five elements which are different vibrations of life energy, and the five tanmatras (five fundamental atoms) which have the same names as the five elemental energies.

There is a chart in Dr. Stone's writings called the Pentamirus combination of the elements (discussed later in this chapter), which is actually the classification of the make-up of the five tanmatras and not, as I originally thought, the five elemental energies. In point of fact you cannot separate the five elements and the five tanmatras. The simplest way I can explain this relationship—and let me hasten to point out that is just my understanding—is that all matter is composed of different fundamental atoms, the five tanmatras, and that each of these atoms is energized by a specific vibratory rate of prana; for example, the earth or prithvi tanmatra is energized by the earth vibration of prana which is distributed throughout the body by the earth chakra. Note that the name for the earth elemental energy is also prithvi. The actual make-up of the earth tanmatra is one half pure earth and the other half equal quantities of the other four atoms, but its basic nature is earthy because that is the quality of life energy that infuses it. When these fundamental atoms become charged with the life energy, they attract each other through polarity and tend to have certain areas of the body where they congregate in great numbers, creating a particular oval field or area of activity, though all are present in varying quantities throughout the body.

With this understanding in mind we can now look at the manipulations in Polarity Therapy as having two different phases. The first, in which we work on the distribution of the elemental energies throughout the body by working on the chakras and the nervous system, and the second phase where we seek to repolarize the different fields of the body so that the energized atoms can attract each other and work harmoniously together. To give an example, suppose a client has a problem with their breathing which is obviously related to their air chakra and the air oval field, so your therapeutic work will be a combination of checking that the air chakra is functioning adequately and distributing its energy throughout the chest to the air tanmatras, and then by polarizing the air oval field, ensuring that the re-energized air tanmatras are then attracting each other and working in harmony.

In a sense, it is impossible to separate the concept of the five elements and the five tanmatras as they both function together, and we could say that all matter is energy anyway. I am not saying that the above model is anything other than a description of a subtle reality that is easy to grasp and work with. Your work must be based upon a clarity of mind that allows you to practice with confidence, even though it is not possible to define reality which is always greater than our ability to conceptualize accurately.

Polarisation

Dr. Stone pointed out that unless the five elements (the energised finer fundamental atoms) within our body are polarized appropriately, we cannot attract the finer essences of matter (the tanmatras) from our diet to replenish our energy fields and thereby maintain our structure. I have found that the model that I have just presented really helped to clarify what Dr. Stone meant when he talked about polarisation and de-polarisation, and how this differs from his discussion of the five rivers of energy. The terms polarisation and de-polarisation relate to the ability of the finer substances to attract their constituent components for balanced functioning. The 'one energy' which is modulated by the chakras is that which activates the finer essences of matter and gives them the ability to attract and repel.

The five different vibrations of prana flow throughout the whole of the body. They are created as a modulation or step down of the primary current of free prana in the atmosphere which we take in by breathing, and which is transferred by the sinuses to the brain. Once the prana is in the brain it is passed down the body via the caduceus currents. In the process of flowing down the body it is modulated at various power stations along the way, the chakras, so as to enable it to perform different functions in the body. The chakras are five different centres of energetic activity that occur down the length of the spinal column, where it is the action of our consciousness that transforms the prana into different vibrations. The chakras are centres of consciousness and energy. When the free prana comes in to the body it is undifferentiated, pure volitionless energy. The action of our consciousness at the chakra centres gives it a quality of volition or mindfulness. In simple terms it knows what it has to do. It is due to the fact that life energy is imbued with consciousness and because it flows in quite different channels from that of our ordinary nervous system that we have the possibility of a full and total perception of the structure of our body at the most subtle essence level of existence. A perception cultivated in many spiritual traditions as the true meaning of the phrase 'man know thyself.'

As our consciousness itself moves through phases of fear and negativity in response to inner self reflections about outer experience conveyed to it by the central nervous system, so the energy from the chakras can be imbued with certain negative or fearful qualities. When the modulated energy from a chakra carries a vibration of negativity with it, it does not polarize the fundamental atoms properly, so physical malfunctioning can often occur. It also creates the basis of the cellular memory. These energy based cellular memories are what is so often activated by a Polarity treatment. What actually happens is that as the fresh energy is brought to an area where the atoms carry this kind of energy based memory, the old stagnant memory-laden energy is displaced and returns to the chakra that created it, and its content is then once more brought back in to conscious awareness.

As the chakras are the medium through which certain qualities of consciousness influence the body, it seems relevant to look at the particular qualities associated with each chakra. The throat chakra qualities, when the consciousness is in balance, are the feelings of humility, reverence and bliss. The sense of actually being a soul. When the consciousness is out of balance then the feeling is one of grief, a loss of connection with the source of all life. At this chakra level the one life energy as manifested by God is changed or modulated the least from its original nature, which indicates that the state of consciousness related to this chakra is that quality of consciousness so sought after in the mystical experience of oneness with the universe, and which functions as spiritual aspiration. The particular quality of the energy is one of space.

The balanced qualities of consciousness at the heart or air chakra level are the soul qualities of love, compassion and imagination. The consciousness when disturbed manifests as desire or wanting things that you do not have, and chasing shadows. At this chakra level the modulation of the one life force functions as the need to relate to others. The particular quality of the energy is mobility.

The qualities of consciousness at the solar plexus or fire chakra are joy and enthusiasm. The sense of self. The feelings at this level when the consciousness is unbalanced is anger, rage and hatred. At this level the modulation of the one life energy is at a point of balance and functions as the need to expand and grow to full self realization. The quality of the energy is heat.

The qualities of consciousness at the sacral or water chakra level are body level feelings, sensitivity, and empathy. The experience of gender. When the consciousness is unbalanced it manifests as gluttony or I want more. The modulation of the one life energy is functioning as racial drives which manifest as the protective instincts. The quality of the energy is smooth and flowing.

The qualities of consciousness associated with the base or earth chakra are possessiveness and sexual desire, when unbalanced consciousness at this level manifests as fear. The modulation of the one energy is ensuring the continuing function in the universe of the one life energy through the creation of new life by the sexual act. The quality of the energy is stability.

The Oval Fields

The five oval fields of the body are five cavities within the body where there are concentrations of various different kinds of activities. The five elements (or the five energized tanmatras) tend to congregate so that the fire element is in the head oval, the ether element in the throat oval, the air element is in the chest oval, the earth element in the abdominal oval and the water element in the pelvic oval (Fig. 4a). All the elements are present throughout the body, but these are the areas in which their physical functioning predominates. The predominant water element position in this chart represents its major physical function, which is reproduction; the earth element position represents digestion; the air element position represents respiration; the ether element represents speech; and, finally, the fire element position represents vision.

CHART NO. 6. PRIMARY FIELDS OF SPACE CIRCLES AS BODY CAVITIES WITH THEIR CROSS OVER POLARITY LINES OF ENERGY AND ONE NEUTER CENTER IN EACH. THE CHEST REPRESENTS THE PHYSICAL FIELD OF AIRINESS AND RESPIRATION. THE ENERGY ASPECT OF THE AIRY ELEMENT IS USUALLY ATTRIBUTED TO THE MIND, THE BRAIN, AND THE NERVOUS SYSTEM, PRIOR TO PHYSICAL FUNCTION.

The fact that there is a different way of labelling the five oval fields has caused more confusion than just about anything else in this book. The location and correspondence of the five ovals as outlined above is the way that most Polarity teachers, practitioners and students understand the five oval fields. It is very clearly a statement about the physical aspect of the function of each of the five elements and where that physical activity is most dominant in the body. When I first studied Polarity I too had just this clear

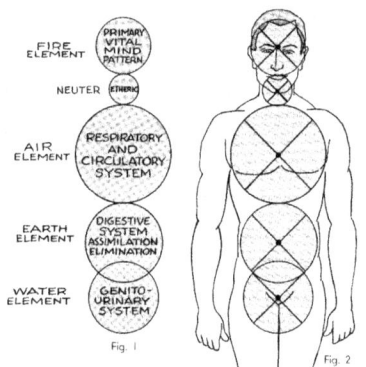

52

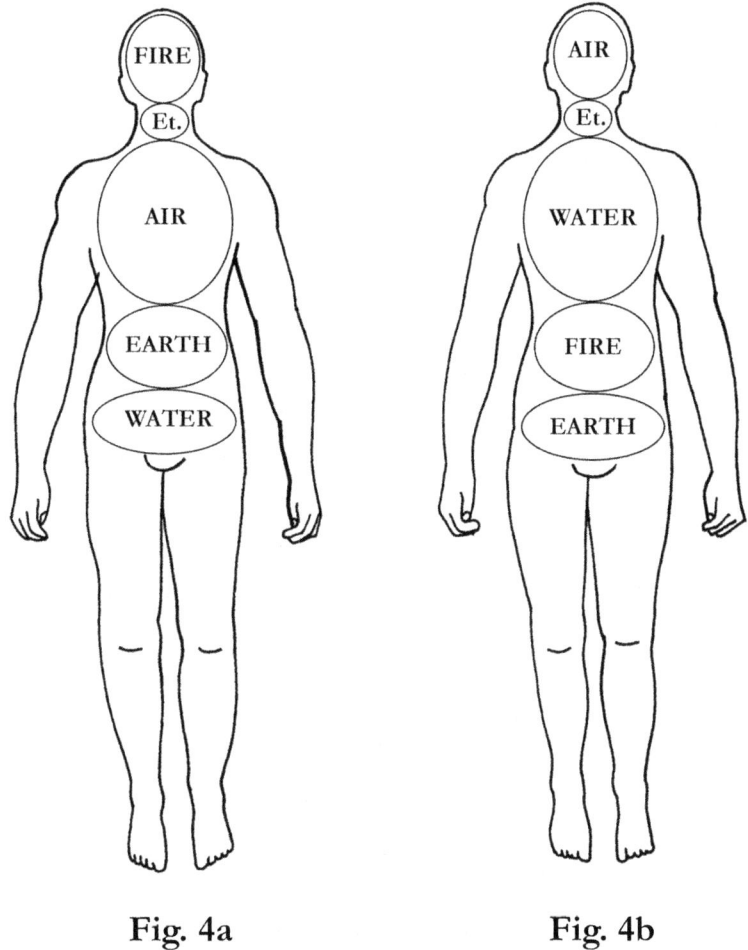

Fig. 4a   **Fig. 4b**

understanding. However, I got thrown into confusion when I studied the chart reproduced opposite to where Dr. Stone discusses the five ovals and their elemental correspondences.

In the second sentence at the top of the chart he wrote: "The chest represents the physical field of airiness and respiration," which made sense to me because this confirmed my understanding of the chest as air. The complexity arose when I noted that the third sentence said: "The energy aspect of the airy element is usually attributed to the mind, the brain and nervous system," which I understood as being true from my study of all the various correspondences attributed to the air element. However, when Dr. Stone differentiated between the physical aspect and the energetic aspect of each element in relation to the ovals, I realised that it was possible to create quite a different labelling from the usual chart. If the reader studies his commentary on the chart, the following will be noted:

> Each field will be recognized in its function, as it is given throughout the book and well illustrated in charts No. 1, 2 and 3 in Book II. Each field has a vibratory keynote of its own as well as specific POLARITY currents for action. The physical aspect of the field is the negative phase. The positive, wireless energy which flows over it is the positive pole in each field. That is why two illustrations are given in this chart.
>
> Vol. I, Book 3, p. 51

The first and most familiar chart of the five oval field correspondences is taken from the physical function aspect of each field, this being the negative phase, as Dr. Stone says above. He goes on to explain that, in Ayurveda, the airy function is also related to the brain and mind, rather than to the fire element, the latter being the usual way in which we label the head in terms of its relationship to the elements. He says it is simply due to one's perspective and whether one is looking at the oval field area on the body from the centre of the field outward or from outside its periphery inward. However, he then goes on to discuss not the five oval fields but the three vital centres, labelling them as 1) the superior (the brain) as being the positive pole representing the airy mind patterns; 2) the middle or neutral pole of the chest being the energy of fire and emotional feeling in the chest; and 3) the pelvis as the negative pole and fluidic or watery essence. This is a description that relates to Chart 2 in the same book where he shows the three vital centres which should not be confused with the five ovals. This sudden shift in topic from discussing the five ovals to the three vital centres is confusing.

It's important to point out that if one is studying Dr. Stone's writings and finds a section that is really difficult to understand, I can almost guarantee that it is because he is lecturing from a different perspective than the one the reader is trying to understand; or that, without indicating it, he has shifted the topic entirely. Having listened to all the audio recordings of his lectures given in seminars between 1956 and 1973, I have no hesitation in saying that, even though he was a Piscean, he also had a very airy nature so that he can flow easily and fluidly from one aspect of a topic to another and then suddenly make a complete airy shift whose occurrence is sometimes hard to even notice, let alone follow.

Returning to the discussion of the oval fields and considering the energetic, rather than physical, function of the five elements in relation to the oval fields: the head is where air energy is most active as constantly moving airy mind patterns. Ether energy is most active in the throat oval as the rainbow bridge, which is the underlying link between all the energies in the body—the communication channel. In the chest water energy manifests as emotions. Fire energy is present in the abdominal oval and is the source of will and motivational drive. Finally, earth energy in the pelvic oval expresses itself as sexual energy (Fig. 4b).

Dr. Stone's writing about the more energetic aspect of the elements and their expression in the five ovals can be contradictory. For example, in relation to the fire element in its more physical aspect, he writes:

> Each circle, as pictured, has a keynote and a special sense which predominates and characterizes its function - five circles, five senses: (see chart No. 2, Book 2.)
>
> 1 - The most outstanding sense in the head is the sense of sight. It is a sensory function with motor power of direction through the mind forces and light waves.
>
> Vol. I, Book 3, p. 52

Hence, he labels the head as the fire oval. However, later in the same section when talking about the energetic aspect of the ovals, he writes:

> 4 - The digestive system is the sustaining function of the body. A fiery energy digests the food, and the abdominal cavity is like a pot.
>
> Vol. I, Book 3, p. 53

To me, this always read more like a physical manifestation of fire in the abdominal area in which it breaks down food into smaller particles, making it available for assimilation into the body. In the first edition of this book I explained the energetic aspect of fire in the abdominal oval as heat. However, I was never entirely happy with this, because heat is a physical phenomenon and not something I see as related to the life energy and consciousness. Now, in 2017, the way I speak of the fiery energy in the abdominal oval is in relation to its function in terms of *will* and *action*. The pit of the stomach, where the fire chakra is located, is also called the solar plexus because of the way so many nerves radiate out from it. It was also described in the early 1900s as *the abdominal brain.*[1] It is the location of the sense of self. A self that is largely invisible, unless it is in action and expressing its will in some way.

Another confusion that arises in relation to the normal oval field labelling (Fig. 4a) is why fields are not more directly linked according to the location of the chakras. It seems to make logical sense to new students of Polarity Therapy to think that, just as the air and ether chakra energies express themselves locally where these two particular qualities of energy are generated, that this should also be true for the fire, water and earth chakra energies. Yet the earth is more active in the abdomen and the fire in the head.

The way I explain this to students is by drawing on the analogy of the national electrical grid of a country. The reality of energy generation is that the most expedient place to generate energy is not necessarily the same place where that energy is going to be used. As an example, most hydroelectric power generating stations are nowhere near centres of population or industry. The energy generated has to be sent via high voltage electrical cables across long distances to get to where it is needed. It is also interesting to note that the manufacturing industry often uses 440 volts, whereas domestic usage is a step down to either 240 or 110 volts.

To me this is more than just an analogy. It is an expression of the hermetic principle of *as within, so without* because a national power grid is nothing less than the external re-creation of the energetic distribution system within the human body. They both share all the same elements: power generating centres, transmission lines, step down transformers and different areas where specific levels of energy are used.

Keeping all this in mind, it makes sense that the energy generated by the fire chakra may well need to be transported to the head where it is most needed to power certain functions or expressions of that fiery energy. Equally, earth energy generated at the base of the spine needs to be transported to the abdomen where it powers a different set of functions. Furthermore, just as some power generating stations are, in fact, near centres of population where that energy is needed, so too in the body a proportion of air, water and ether energy is used exactly where it is generated.

1. *The Solar Plexus: Abdominal Brain* by, Theron Q. Dumont, 1918, Advanced Thought Publishing Company Chicago.

Oval Field Treatment

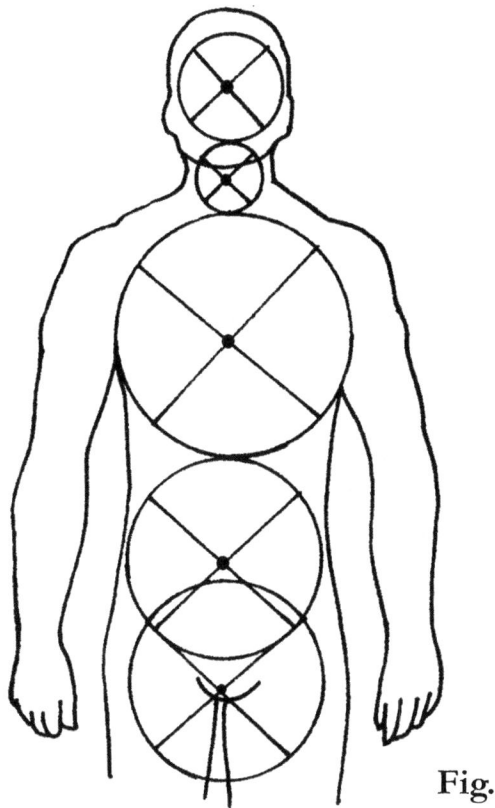

Fig. 5

You can balance any individual element by working on the appropriate oval field in the body using bi-polar contacts. To do this you have to imagine each field as a three-dimensional structure with a central point. To polarize any sore or blocked area in the field you make proportional contacts based on the distance of the blocked area to the central point. What this means is you imagine a line from a sore point through the centre of the field continuing on to an equidistant point on the other side. You then stimulate each point alternately until the blockage is cleared.

For example, when working the fire oval in the head a sore point on the middle of the occipital base near the foramen magnum will have a corresponding release point on the middle to upper part of the forehead, in line with but above the third eye area. As all contacts made following this rule are diagonal contacts, you are stimulating the deep caduceus energy currents in the body. This concept is illustrated in two-dimensional form in Fig. 5.

It is possible to balance any two elements and their manifestation in the oval fields by using bi-polar contacts, one on the area of function of one of the elements in question, and the other on the area of function of the other element. This concept can be utilized when dealing with imbalances in the physical aspect of elemental function or the energetic. For example, in the Tummy Rock[2] you will see that it is a balancing of the fire and water Elements (the left-hand contact on the head representing the fire element in its physical area of manifestation, the right hand on the pelvis representing the water element in its area of physical manifestation). If you look at the technique and the contact areas

2. *Polarity Therapy Healing with Life Energy,* by Alan Siegel M.S. N.D. and Phil Young, p. 35.

from an energetic viewpoint it is a balancing of the air and earth elements (air relating to the head and earth relating to the pelvis).

Most Polarity techniques that are done on the central vertical axis of the body with the hands separated by a distance of at least ten inches or 25 cm will be a balancing of two or more elements. A contact on the chest combined with one just below the diaphragm could be considered to be a balancing of the air and earth elements, if we look at the contact areas in terms of the physical manifestation of the elements, looked at energetically the same two contacts would be a balancing of water (chest) and fire (the oval field beneath the diaphragm). This one technique could have a balancing effect on four elements at the same time.

Another example is the coccyx treatment,[3] in which the ganglion of impar is balanced against muscular tensions in the buttocks, could be said to be a balancing of earth, air, fire, and water. This is clear when you realize that the coccyx is the physical location of the earth chakra (earth), and is the location of the negative pole of the sympathetic nervous system, the ganglion of impar (fire). Looking at the buttocks we see that they are the physical motor pole of the water element. The buttock area is also a contact area for the para-sympathetic nervous system in that the sacral nerves are influenced (air), and in a general sense the treatment also affects the cerebrospinal impulses (air). Once again four elements are being balanced.

Elemental Treatment Strategy

Dr. Stone wrote that any energy block is by definition, in its inception, a disturbance of the air element. The energy has stopped moving. The problem can be resolved quickly by working fire and water simultaneously. Working fire and water together will create a lot of air (or steam, to be exact) that will push through the blockage. However, this will not work if the blockage has become crystallized, as you would then be trying to resolve an earth element problem. Different elements would require stimulating and balancing. From this it is obvious that you should not just be considering balancing an element when it is disturbed by only working on it in isolation, but be looking at the secondary effects of working two elements simultaneously as possibly being a far more effective route.

If you were treating an acute fire problem, which of the following approaches would be best? Stimulating water and relating it to fire, as water controls fire; stimulating earth in relation to fire, so that the fire is suffocated; stimulating ether to space the fire out, so that it loses its concentrated power? What about cross-balancing earth and air, making

3. *Polarity Therapy Healing with Life Energy,* by Alan Siegel M.S. N.D. and Phil Young, p. 124.

stimulating contacts on the earth and satvic contacts on the air, thereby using earth to suffocate the fire, at the same time as you are calming and balancing the air that is fuelling the fire? What would be the most effective approach? Unfortunately, there are no rules that will help you. You just have to follow your intuition for each individual client. Always be flexible in your approach and do not be afraid to change your tack in the middle of a treatment.

Another aspect to elemental interaction is that a problem manifesting as a significant disturbance in one element may actually have its source in some level of disturbance in one or more of the others. In this case, you may need to balance both elements in one session by firstly working on the element that is most disturbed and then addressing the disturbance in the other element. Alternatively, you could balance both elements simultaneously. As an example: in diaphragm releasing manipulations in which one hand is placed on the shoulder and the other hand is working out any tenderness in the buttocks, you are balancing the air and water elements, the air element being represented in the shoulder contact (air element triad: shoulders, kidneys, ankles) and the water element represented in the buttock contact (water element triad: breasts, genitals, feet—the buttocks being the posterior motor positive pole of the genitals). In general, you can work any of the areas of correspondence (chakra, oval field, astrological triad, elemental reflexes) of one element to those of the other. Many variations are possible e.g. balance the oval field or chakra of one element to the astrological triad of the other to balance them both. You could also cross-balance the two sets of astrological triads and so forth.

The only thing that will precisely define the effect of any elemental treatment is where your mental intention lies; clarify that and your work will become specific to the balance between the particular elements that will be of most benefit to the client. Balancing any individual element is important, but we must remember that they do not exist in isolation, so learn to use the technique outlined above. Study the way that you work. What are you actually doing? What is your intention?

Having been a student for many years of both the Western and Eastern traditions of esoteric philosophy, and more recently of the oceanic cultures of the Pacific, I have yet to come across anything even remotely approaching a definitive system. All schools of thought have their good points and their weak points. I myself have worked with a number of other approaches to the energy balancing work apart from the five elements, everything from a mind energy model to a transpersonal approach that transcends concepts of dualism, to the four-principle approach. All these strategies are valid and it is my feeling that our ultimate goal as healers is to transcend all the various models, which are in their very nature incomplete, to a direct knowingness of the fundamentals of life and energy.

The Pentamirus Combination of the 5 Elements

These twenty five pentamirus combinations are the elemental makeup of a number of different aspects of the human being.

The **Ether** combinations are **Emotions**

Grief is the principle quality of ether, a feeling of nothingness. Desire is produced by a combination of air and ether. Anger is a combination of fire and ether. Attachment (or greed) is a combination of water and ether. Fear is a combination of earth and ether. The relationship of the emotions to the ether element is clear if we realize that an emotion is a movement of energy or feeling in the body to which we ascribe a specific thought or value judgement. A feeling only becomes an emotion when it reaches our conscious awareness by passing through the throat area, both for recognition and evaluation at a mental level, but also because it is only when a feeling reaches this level in the body that we can emote it, that is express it or bring it out.

The **Air** combinations are **Qualities of Movement**

Speed (mobility) is the principle quality of air. Lengthening is a combination of ether and air. Shaking is a combination of fire and air. Motion (slow movement) is a combination of water and air. Contraction is a combination of earth and air. The relationship of air to certain qualities of movement is obvious, one only has to study nature or your own body, the shaking and shivering of our bodies to warm up when cold (air/fire), and how lethargic we feel on a humid day when the air is laden with water, for example.

The **Fire c**ombinations are **Physiological Drives** or **Motivations**

Hunger is the main quality of fire. Sleep is a combination of ether and fire. Thirst is a combination of air and fire. Lust(re) is a combination of water and fire. Laziness is a combination of earth and fire. The fire combinations are all physiological drives, the need to eat, sleep, drink, have sex and relax. Air and fire are quite capable of drying out water, making you thirsty. Ether is capable of spacing out the fiery mental activity, making you sleep.

The **Water** combinations are **Bodily Fluids**

Semen is the main quality of water. Saliva is a combination of ether and water. Sweat is a combination of air and water. Urine is a combination of fire and water. Blood is a combination of earth and water. The water combinations are all bodily fluids. Saliva (or mucus) being produced in bodily cavities (ether). Sweat being produced by movement (air).

The **Earth** combinations are **Bodily Tissues**

Bones are the principle quality of earth. Hair is a combination of ether and earth. Skin is a combination of air and earth. Blood vessels are a combination of fire and earth. Flesh is a combination of water and earth. The earth combinations are all solid matter in the body. Skin is earth and air because it breathes and eliminates, flesh is water and earth because of its semi-solid sponge-like quality and all the various fluids that it contains.

Some of the reasoning behind certain of the combinations is not always clear but they will become clear if you think them through carefully. A knowledge of the combinations can be an invaluable tool when trying to discover the root causes in elemental terms of various physical problems.

Pentamirus Treatment

In terms of working with the pentamirus combinations, the possibilities are myriad. As an example, if a client is struggling with insomnia you would review the pentamirus combinations to see what information they can give you. Sleep is the result of the interaction between ether as the subsidiary and fire as the dominant element. The ether energy has the effect of modulating the fire, in this case, spacing it out. So, the client needs work on the fire and ether elements.

The approach I would commonly use to bring balance between the ether and fire elements, in relation to this pentamirus combination, is to work at the chakra level. I do this in two phases. In the first phase, I place thc fingers of my left hand lightly over the throat (ether chakra) and place my right hand, palm down, over the solar plexus area (fire chakra). I then, either satvically hold both places, or use gentle alternating rajasic technique. Then I change sides on the table and place the fingers of the right hand on the throat and the left hand on the solar plexus stimulating and holding as appropriate. Energetically, this is creating a type of circular flow to and from each chakra, as well as balancing their interaction.

For the second phase, I simultaneously stimulate both big toes (ether) and then both thumbs (left/right balancing). Then I connect the thumb and big toe on each side using alternate stimulation (top/bottom balancing) before connecting the thumbs and big toes on each side to the solar plexus (fire chakra) using alternate rajasic stimulation and then satvic holding.

As another example, if a client has a lot of contraction in their body and limitation of movement this would be viewed, in terms of the penatmirus combinations, as an imbalance in the interaction of earth with air. When I suggest that the way to resolve this would be to work with these two elements, most students question the concept, often saying, "Won't this make the contraction worse?" It is an understandable concern, because if contraction is caused by the interaction of earth with air surely working on these two elements will just create more contraction?

They key lies in realising that all the interactions in the 25 pentamirus combinations are natural. Contraction is an important action in the body, particularly in terms of organ function. The key, as ever, is balance. We need contraction, but not too much. By working both elements using Polarity techniques, a more balanced interaction is always created.

It is also quite common for students to look at the air pentamirus combinations and notice that lengthening, which is the opposite of contraction, is created by the interaction of ether with air. They then ask why it would not be better to work on the ether and air balance to resolve the contraction issue.

This way of working with the elements, which we explored earlier, is based upon the general concept of elemental interaction whereby one looks to the action of a different element to resolve an imbalance. Working with the water element to resolve a disturbance in the fire element is a classic example of this type of balancing. This is, perhaps, by far the most common way elemental treatment strategy is taught. However, this approach is sometimes ineffective, mostly because it does not address what Dr. Stone called an energetic 'lock.' This is a very common condition, particularly in chronic cases which, pragmatically speaking, form the bulk of our practise, whereby the energy in any element becomes locked up in a particular pattern either physically, energetically and/or mentally. In this situation, if there is a lock in fire, no amount of water element work will be effective simply because the fire is locked and unresponsive. The best way to deal with this situation, putting it both colloquially and literally, is to fight fire with fire. In this case, you work directly with the client's fire element, stimulating and balancing it directly, to break the lock. Once the lock is released the fire will, of course, settle and balance within itself, as well as become responsive to the effects of the other elements.

The Four Principles

The Four Principles is an interesting way of looking at the human body and human behaviour. They are by name, the Thinking, the Going, the Doing, and the Being Principle. Each principle relates to a kind of activity. Activities which are common to all of us at various times and to different degrees. They each relate to a specific area of the human body and to specific energy patterns. It is possible to characterize any of your clients by the balance of the four principles that they manifest. It is also easy to see which of the principles is being over or under used. Then use this understanding to clarify the kind of energy balancing techniques that would be most appropriate for them. It is important to realize that the balance of the four principles will vary over a period of time. They are not fixed in any way, nor are we seeking to create some kind of perfect balance between their usage by the client. What we want is that they have the ability to flow easily from expressing one principle into another.

The Thinking Principle

The Thinking Principle is simply the amount of thinking that a person does; the degree to which they use their conscious mind, their rationality. It is obviously true that some of us do more thinking than others and that we vary from day to day in the amount of rational, analytical thinking that we indulge in. It is also true that some people do very little thinking; that they come from a much more visceral, emotional base. I am sure we have all come across the client who says they do not think; that they are too stupid, silly or childish to be able to think something through. This is rarely the case unless they have some form of serious abnormality of the brain. Everybody is capable of thinking. It would be impossible to survive without the ability to think things through, though it would certainly be true to say that some of us are more adept at it than others. Thinking is an ability that can be developed and sharpened by any of us if we so wish.

Physically, the Thinking Principle relates to the head area. Energetically, it relates to the fire chakra and the fire triad, and the posterior aspect of the umbilical spiral. As soon as a client indicates any kind of a problem with their head, from headaches to spots, look for some kind of an imbalance in their Thinking Principle. Explore their attitudes to their own thinking capabilities. Do they find themselves getting stuck with repetitive patterns of thoughts? Do they think they are stupid? Do they spend vast amounts of time in self reflection and self analysis? There are many other questions you could ask. Why not do a little exploration of your own Thinking Principle as a way of familiarizing yourself with the concept?

The Going Principle

The Going Principle is a person's ability to move, to get up and go. The ability to change position in life. It is linked to the Thinking Principle because the ability to move in life has ramifications beyond the mere physical action of moving the body. Movement is a motor activity that is in the first instance often initiated by the mind. However, it is also true that movement can be initiated by basic survival mechanisms. These in themselves have little or nothing to do with conscious thought processes. When looking at a client's Going Principle not only are you going to be investigating their physical mobility and strength, but also looking at their ability to change their life situations, i.e. relationships, occupation/etc. For any movement to occur there must be good contact with a stable base (the earth) to push off from. Check the contact that their feet make with the ground. A stable inner centre of gravity is also an important requirement before one can initiate effective movement. Look at their self image. How strong and accurate is that?

Physically the Going Principle relates to the pelvis, legs, and feet. Energetically it relates to the fire, water, and earth chakras, their associated astrological triads, and the posterior aspect of the umbilical spiral. If a client has any problems in the lower half of the body, from the pelvis down to the feet, then you are looking for an imbalance in the Going Principle. Even sexual problems are linked to problems in the Going Principle, but rather than tell you the connection see if you can think it out for yourself!

The Doing Principle

The Doing Principle is directly related to a person's motivation. Do they get things done in life? How good are they at achieving the things they want to do? Once again it is linked to both the Thinking Principle and the Going Principle, as any action is first a process of ideation, and then a movement towards the manifestation of the idea ('I am going to do it'), and finally the process of actually doing it. We all do things or we try and achieve something through our efforts. Doing and effort are for most people fundamentally related. If you are going to do something then it will require a certain amount of effort. Unfortunately few people realize that the more effort they make, very often the less they actually achieve. The amount of effort a person puts into a project is related to their ability to maintain sufficient motivation to see it through to its completion. The more effort it takes the harder it is to stay motivated, whereas the more gracefully and economically they can apply their energy the easier it is to see something through to its completion. The Doing Principle is therefore both a person's ability to 'do' things and their ability to see their actions through to a satisfactory completion.

Physically the Doing Principle relates to the middle and upper back, neck, shoulders, arms and hands. Energetically it relates to the ether, air and fire chakras, their associated astrological triads and the joints of the upper body. It also relates to the posterior aspect of the umbilical spiral. Does a client ever complete anything, do they use their energy efficiently, do they even begin a project or are they always going to do it but never quite begin to act? Negative answers to these questions all point to a disturbance of the doing principle.

The Being Principle

The Being Principle is very simply a person's ability to 'be,' it is a tranquil inner space in which there is no volitional activity, a space in which to experience the effects of your actions and as such it is the final phase of a movement that begins with the Thinking Principle. It is the point in any activity where a person absorbs and self reflects upon their emotional and physical movements within the world. It is also the point at which learning takes place. The balanced manifestation of the Being Principle allows the sense of completion to become a part of a person's life. In some sense when we are simply being we are in touch with our own personal experience of God. To be able to 'do' effectively one must be able to 'be,' but there has to be a balance between these two principles. People who are compulsively doing things rarely ever experience any satisfaction in their doingness because they never take time to self reflect, and people who are always just being never experience the joy of creativity.

Physically the Being Principle relates to the abdomen and front of the chest. Energetically it relates to the anterior aspect of the umbilical spiral, the five-pointed star and the long straight line currents of energy. A client manifesting an imbalance in their Being Principle will often experience problems with their vitality. Ascertaining a client's attitude towards such things as rest and relaxation can tell you much about their relationship to their Being Principle. Do they use prayer or meditation in their daily life, and do they regularly take stock of their lives? Do they allow themselves the time to experience the glow of satisfaction that comes after a job well done?

It should be obvious that the Four Principles can be related to the Five Elements, and an exploration of their possible inter-relationships can prove to be extremely illuminating.

6. Mind and Energy

Mind is the finest substance of matter operating in three bodies as three fields of consciousness:

The causal body is the pattern field of the mind; here it is the ideal or superconscious mind;

In the etheric and emotional field, mind operates thru [through] the senses. It is the normal conscious mind;

In the gross physical body, mind governs all involuntary functions and repairs. It operates as the subconscious mind.

Vol. I, Book 2, p. 3

In the above quote from Dr. Stone's writings he classifies mind as being triune in nature. He divides it into three levels, sub-conscious, conscious and higher conscious. What are the energy patterns that relate to each level of consciousness? Some might ask whether this is even a viable question. It is my belief that there are different energy patterns that relate directly to each level of mind. I believe that it would be true to say that perhaps seventy-five percent of the techniques that Dr. Stone developed work on the energy patterns relating to the sub-conscious mind; the realm of feelings and the force behind the repair and maintenance functions of the body. Specifically, these energy patterns are the five bi-lateral long-line currents, the five lower chakras, the east-west currents and the caduceus currents. Any work on these energy patterns can be considered to be working with the client's sub-conscious mind.

The Sub-conscious Mind

It is the sub-conscious mind that supervises all the repair work in the body. It holds all the basic survival mechanisms, as well as being the storehouse of the memory. It is the sub- conscious mind that gives us the sensations of energy flow in the body, the feelings that eventually become emotions when they are linked to certain thoughts by the conscious mind. My concept of the sub-conscious mind is that it is a creature of habit. It likes patterns, particularly stable ones, and it is also remarkably stubborn. I see its basic function as the maintenance of patterns. It would be a very difficult life if we had to consciously maintain the physiological functioning of our body. Can you imagine what it would be like to have to consciously keep your heart beating; if every breath had to be conscious; if you had to direct the whole digestive process as well as attending to all the necessary repair work in the body? The sub-conscious does all these things for us. To do these tasks effectively it must store a vast number of patterns. These patterns contain extremely detailed information on the functioning of the body. The sub-conscious is constantly matching body function to these patterns, much like a computer system runs an executive programme to maintain its basic functioning capabilities.

The sub-conscious mind is also able to learn new patterns with remarkable ease. Patterns that do not just relate to behavioural patterns or practical skills but that also relate to altered patterns of physiological functioning. This basic ability is one that we use all the time in our everyday lives. The classic example is learning to drive a car. This is an activity that has to be studied consciously with great attention to detail in its initial stages until we have learned the patterns of behaviour needed to do it effectively. These patterns are at a certain point then shifted to the sub-conscious mind, which stores them and enacts them whenever we require access to that particular skill, leaving our conscious mind free to attend to other matters. In the case of driving a car we all know when this has happened because suddenly we have sufficient free conscious attention to be able to hold a conversation and drive fluidly at the same time. The same process occurs as we grow up. We are taught certain patterns of behaviour by the adults around us which in the course of time become sub-conscious patterns that we use automatically. These kind of learned patterns form the basis of our character.

Once a pattern has been stored the sub-conscious mind will in general hold on to it indefinitely. Patterns which relate to physical functioning are normally held with greater tenacity than patterns which relate to behaviours, but as all patterns have survival value on some level this distinction is not always valid. The sub-conscious mind uses all the different patterns held within the memory as the blueprint for modulating the flow of energy and consciousness in the body. It is these patterns which determine the volume and direction of energy flow that underlie the physical and emotional structure of the body. In any trauma where distortion of the physical structure occurs the energy flow becomes distorted, which instantly shows up in the sub-conscious as a pattern disruption. This in turn sets in motion the basic survival mechanism, whereby the sub-conscious mind will begin to manipulate the energy until it again matches the appropriate pattern stored in the memory, so that healing at the physical level can take place.

In some case where the physical damage is too great or if there are other behavioural patterns of a conflicting nature being activated, then chronic unresolvable energetic imbalances will result and no physical healing will occur. For example, a client falls injuring their knee. In normal circumstances the sub-conscious will rebalance the energy and healing will begin, but if at this particular time in their personal life they are experiencing a definite lack of attention from their partner, and should they have stored a behavioural pattern to the effect that they receive a lot of attention when ill or incapacitated in some way, the net result is going to be that both patterns are going to be activated simultaneously and the sub-conscious is not going to be able to rebalance the energy due to the conflicting nature of each pattern. The need of the attention pattern in this case will override the basic healing pattern. The conflict will only resolve itself if the needs of the attention pattern become satisfied, which in turn will depend on the responses of the client's partner. This kind of resolution will not always occur, particularly if the relationship between the client and their partner was fundamentally damaged before the accident. The required increase in attention will not, in all probability, happen and the attention pattern will continue to block the healing. To resolve this kind of situation some form of outside therapeutic intervention is needed to help to de-activate the attention pattern.

All long-standing illness, disease and energetic imbalance can be thought of as a conflict of patterns in the sub-conscious mind. In this situation you are going to have to work diligently not only to get the energy unblocked and flowing freely, but to work simultaneously with the client to get them to realize that they have some underlying behavioural pattern that is preventing them from recovering. In psychological terms these health negating behavioural patterns are the basis of the phenomena known as *secondary gain*. When working with a client to discover the nature of their patterns of secondary gain remember that it can sound as if you are saying that they *want* to be ill, which at a conscious level is hardly ever true. If you do not contextualize what you are saying you will create a great deal of very conscious, fiery resistance and probably lose the client as well. A situation that serves no one. You must give them an understanding of the nature of the sub-conscious mind, that what it does is always out of our conscious awareness.

Interestingly a 'habit pattern' can occur as the result of a long-standing conflict between a healing pattern and one that is negating it. Sometimes the behavioural pattern that was negating the healing pattern can have long since become inactive, but if this took a long time, say in excess of a few months, a third pattern can be set up. This would be a simple habit pattern which in effect is saying 'illness is my normal state of being.' If you have given a client a series of sessions and they do not seem to be improving, it does not necessarily mean that you have been doing the wrong thing or that your energy release work has been ineffective. It is more likely that you are being thwarted by a very deeply entrenched behavioural pattern. It is at this point that you must begin to work very directly with the sub-conscious mind patterns through deep analysis, affirmation work, or give them a good "Dutch uncle talk," to use Dr. Stone's phrase. Your approach is probably going to have to be very dynamic and fiery, but you must have the client's trust for this to work.

The reason that affirmations and the fiery Dutch uncle approach works is because one of the other basic qualities of the sub-conscious mind is its childlike impressionability. As a Polarity therapist you have the edge over many other therapeutic approaches because you deal with life energy, which is the essence of real magic. After all you can create the most amazing sensations of movement, heat, and vibration in the body sometimes without even touching it. Even though the sub-conscious mind works with energy its own understanding of the laws which govern its action are often quite limited, particularly in the understanding that it can be influenced so readily and directly by someone else. However, the sub- conscious mind learns very quickly! In a sense, it seems to me that these behavioural patterns are intelligent, as individual segments of consciousness (or unconsciousness) that in some way have the capability to self regulate and adapt through a feedback mechanism. This is why the first two or perhaps three Polarity sessions can be so effective, and why it can get more difficult as the sessions continue. Not as some people think because you are having to work more deeply, but because you are dealing with a very much more knowledgeable sub-conscious. You could say that the first couple of sessions slip in beneath the defences because the sub-conscious patterns of secondary gain do not understand the nature of the enemy. To be able to maintain the therapeutic progress you as therapist-magician must have new spells to introduce as the therapy continues, and the artistry to come up with new and different ways to work with the life energy. As a Polarity therapist it is reassuring to know that you can approach the work in so many different ways through touch, diet, exercise and counseling. As Dr. Stone himself did, there is even the possibility of using precious metals and crystals. Magic indeed!

In Polarity Therapy two of the basic principles are the Hermetic laws, *as above, so below* and *as within, so without*. In reading over the last few pages on the sub-conscious mind you will have noticed the allusion I made to the similarity between the sub-conscious mind and a computer system, and, in fact, I do believe there is a strong relationship between the two. I suspect the ability to create the computers we use today comes from the fact that our sub-conscious mind is the computer within, which we have now manifested as the electronic silicon-chip machines without. Indeed, how could we create something outside of ourselves that was not somehow already within us in some form or another?

As Polarity therapists we are working to unblock the flow of life energy so that the healing patterns can work effectively. We do not need to decide in what way the energy should flow. It is the fundamental healing patterns stored in the memory of the sub-conscious mind that will determine that. However, we do need to have an awareness of all the things that might prevent those patterns from being effective. An understanding of the nature and functioning of the sub-conscious mind is invaluable for both yourself and your clients. Polarity therapy is as much a learning process for the client as it is a healing one. All Polarity practitioners are health educators as well as therapists.

The Conscious Mind

The nature of the conscious mind is quite different from that of the sub-conscious mind. The conscious mind is composed of all the psychological processes that you can be or are aware of. For example, your sense perceptions of both your body and the world around you and your ability to reason. It does not function independently of the sub-conscious mind. It relies on the sub-conscious to provide it with access to memory. Memories not just of earlier life experiences but memories concerning the manner in which the conscious sense perceptions and information about life absorbed at a conscious level can be processed. If we look at the computer analogy again then the sub-conscious mind is the data and programmes, and the conscious mind is the central processing unit; that part of the computer that processes, manipulates and modifies input or new data on the basis of pre-existing patterns. It absorbs the new information and holds it in the short-term memory (RAM). It also accesses stored programmes and data from the long-term memory and places them in the short-term memory. Then having both the new information and a pattern as to how it can be processed in the short-term memory, it manipulates or modifies the new information on the basis of this pattern.

As human beings we take in information and then manipulate it in various ways based on previous experience, and we call this 'thinking.' The way in which we think is based on previous experience and learning. Most of our thinking is done on the basis of patterns that are frequently referred to as beliefs. Our biggest problem is that we do not review and modify our patterns of information processing—*our beliefs*—often enough. We end up spending an inordinate amount of time on what is best described as distorted thinking; that is thinking that is inappropriate to our current life situation. This happens because most of us do not actually learn from our experience, as learning is not experiencing life and thinking about those experiences with a pattern of logic that was appropriate ten years ago. It is absorbing life experience and allowing this to modify our actual patterns of thinking. In computer terminology this is analogous to the point at which there is a recognition that the kind of information that you are having to deal with now requires a new programme that has greater built-in flexibility and power. A programme that is able to deal more adequately with the new input. In a computer system, if you input too much new information or information of a different nature from that which the programme is able to process, it will crash. It will just stop functioning. In a sense it is rather unfortunate that as human beings we are not as limited as a computer system. We have an *enormous* capacity for absorbing new experience and processing it by inappropriate beliefs before we crash. It can take us an amazing length of time before realizing that there is a problem.

Distorted thinking on the basis of outmoded beliefs is a major therapeutic problem. How many times have you heard a client make such statements as "I am always ill", "my relationships never work; "nobody likes me," "I never have any money," "you wont be able to help me," "my husband (wife) does not understand me," "I am worthless," "I never succeed at anything," "I can"t change my job," "doing that will not help." All these and many more that you hear every day are all examples of rigidity and distortion in the conscious mind. Always suspect distorted thinking when a client uses words like; can't, never, always, nobody. Words that imply limitation and negativity. You can always ascertain the amount of sub-conscious holding on when working with a client to alter their way of thinking, by the degree of passion and emotionality with which they defend their old beliefs. As we all know, some beliefs are easily changed in the light of clearer logic or new experience, but I am sure you have all had experience of trying to change some aspect of yourself and your thinking in your own personal therapy and met a solid wall of emotional resistance which tells you that it is a pattern which your sub-conscious believes still has survival value.

Affirmations are a basic tool that can be used to change distorted patterns of thinking. I tend to think of them as new programmes for the mind-computer, as the affirmational process is in essence a re-programming technique. If we look at the structure of affirmations the first thing you will notice is that they are always stated in positive terms. Secondly, they are always phrased so as to be the opposite of an old belief. Thirdly, the constant internal repetition and the seeding of your environment with slips of paper with the affirmation written on them, creates a constant input of the new information to the conscious mind. It becomes memory resident, a piece of information that is always present in the short-term memory. Ultimately, because of this, it will be a modifying factor when the old belief is activated. In the long term it will be stored in the sub-conscious along with the old belief as a new parameter that will mean the old belief is now always modified when accessed, or that it will modify the old belief so much that it no longer exists in its original form.

Affirmations work best when you can inspire in the client a strong positive attitude towards the technique. This enlists the help of the sub-conscious mind. The best approach to getting a client to feel positive whilst doing the affirmations is to talk passionately about the possibilities that could open up in their life as a result of the changes in their attitudes and thinking. When teaching affirmations there is a real need for you to be positive all the time, even if the results are not manifesting for the client. Even if the final outcome is not the kind of change in the client's outer world as implicit in the technique, it is always possible to emphasize to them the positive internal attitudinal change that always occurs if you do an affirmation for any length of time. At the very least the expectant, hopeful attitude engendered is an excellent result.

In relation to illness and disease the conscious mind has an interesting role. In particular the aspect we call 'awareness' or conscious recognition. A person goes into therapy because they have a conscious awareness that they have a problem. They are aware either of pain and limited mobility or some form of emotional distress. There are of course certain kinds of diseases that do not impinge on conscious awareness until they are at quite an advanced stage, but this situation does not concern us here. As soon as one has an awareness of a problem it creates a response in your thinking. You evaluate your awareness of the problem against your previous experiences of a similar nature to see what you know about it, and to decide if it warrants further attention other than waiting for the body to heal itself or the emotions to calm down. If the problem persists for more than a short period of time your awareness of it will form the experience into a pattern to be stored in your long-term memory. Once this has happened the problem has already become a part of your ongoing reality. This is one reason why during a treatment, if I happen to press on a part of the client's body that is extremely tender, of which they were previously unaware, I pass off the almost inevitable questions of "what is that?," "what does that mean?," or "what does that relate to?," with something like the following response: "it is nothing, just a sore muscle," "it is not important and it does not relate to anything," "it's just a bit of local tension." I do not want them to start worrying about other problems that were out of their awareness. Such worrying only makes them more difficult to resolve. If it is a problem that is out of their awareness just treat it along with the problem that they are aware of.

Memory

It is obvious from our look at mind and energy so far that memory plays a vital role. This role is nicely illustrated by a study done some years ago on people with chronic back trouble, people who said that they experienced almost constant pain. Firstly they found that in actual fact they were not in pain all the time but that sometimes were quite unaware of it. Secondly, if you asked them about the pain at a time when they were not actually feeling it, they would place their hand on their back and re-evoke the experience of the pain from memory. I see memory as a separate entity from mind. It is a separate storehouse for both inner and outer life experiences. Memory can be accessed by all the different levels of mind. Our whole identity is based upon memory. We are the sum of all our previous thoughts and experiences. A great deal of the fragmentation of character and identity that we experience is caused because we can only access a limited proportion of our total life experience at any one time. Many disease states and general imbalance are prolonged due to the client consciously accessing their memory concerning the particular problem. Part of the process of recovery is to no longer re-evoke your memory of the problem. It is quite a common experience for a client to say, in response to your question concerning how they feel about the problem that you have been treating them for, that they were not aware of it so it must be getting better. In part this is due to the fact that quite probably they are in fact getting better, but that also they are no longer interested or even able to access their memory of the discomfort that they felt.

The concept of awareness and memory that I have outlined above is perhaps most simply elucidated in the following situation. A teenager who has had facial spots for some months will wash their face at night and perhaps apply some form of skin treatment before retiring, in the hope that the treatment will remove the spots. When they wake up in the morning it is quite possible that their skin may have cleared significantly, but because this has not happened in the previous weeks they have built up a belief that has become stored in their memory that the spots will probably still be there in the morning. As they lie in bed before either touching their face or looking in the mirror they are often caught up in a number of conflicting thoughts; a hopeful belief that the spots may be gone because the doctor or therapist had said that they would probably take some weeks to go, and a conflicting fearful one based upon weeks of experiencing little or no change every time they look in the mirror. In this situation memory is both supporting and negating the healing process. The question is, which of the thoughts is being enacted by the sub-conscious mind, as that will determine the actual situation. There is always the involvement of the sub-conscious and conscious minds as well as memory in all disease and imbalance.

The pattern of energy that relates directly to the conscious mind is the spirals of energy that radiate from the umbilicus. Dr. Stone called this particular energy pattern 'evolutionary energy' because it is the conscious mind that is the aspect of mind that is constantly seeking new experience and growth. The pattern of energy is a constantly expanding spiral which is but a reflection of the nature of the conscious mind, which is itself always seeking expansion, a broadening of its horizons. As all disease and imbalance involves some form of conscious awareness and distorted thinking, there is always going to be some degree of disturbance in the umbilical spirals of energy. As I pointed out, the sub-conscious and conscious minds work together, it is important to establish a functioning balance between the energy patterns that relate to the sub-conscious mind and those of the conscious mind. This can be done by tying in the umbilical spirals of energy to the chakra system.

There is a challenge in Dr. Stone's writings in that, in his first book, he speaks of there being two centres of fire energy, one in the solar plexus and the other at the navel. In his later books he just speaks of one fire centre, this being the manipura chakra that he located at the navel. Later still, in his *25 Evolutionary Energy Charts*, he speaks of the umbilical centre (the nabhi in Sanskrit) in quite a different way to the earlier books.

I believe, that the umbilical energy centre is not synonymous with the fire or manipura chakra. I see the fire centre or chakra as part of the caduceus system, the source of whose energy is the post birth breath and prana. My personal experience is that it is physically located at the solar plexus.

The umbilical centre, or nabhi, I believe, draws in a specific higher frequency of prana directly from the energy that surrounds us all the time. In the womb, this energy comes from mother via the umbilical cord and creates the physical body. When we are born and the umbilical cord is cut, the umbilical centre begins to draw in energy directly from our greater mother, the Earth. Throughout the rest of an individual's life it continues to function creatively through the conscious mind rather than the physical body.

I do understand both the fire chakra and the navel as being fiery centres. I see the umbilical energy as being both a pre- and post-birth evolutionary fire energy. A *cosmic* creative fire. I view the manipura chakra as a step down of this cosmic fire into a *personal* creative fire. You could think of these two centres as expressing different octaves of fire energy.

The Super-conscious Mind

The super-conscious mind is that aspect of mind that is fundamentally linked to, or is synonymous with, the soul. It is the organizing or seed pattern. In our analogy of the mind as a computer the super-conscious mind is the actual operator, the person who chose the system in the first place and who ultimately determines the input. In my experience the only disease states that are related to the super-conscious mind are major or life threatening illnesses such as cancer. If a person indulges in excessive amounts of distorted thinking and does not adequately utilize the learning capabilities that they have, and refuses to seek out the true meaning of life, from the operator's point of view the information they put in is being badly processed. At a certain point the operator is going to get so frustrated by the computer's inability to deal appropriately with the input that the only choice he has is to shut down the system. He would then either restart the system in the hopes that it was just a temporary bug, or would have to consider creating a completely new programme with which to process the input, but this would mean deleting the old programme.

In human terms, sometimes the only way to shift somebody from such an inappropriate approach to life is that they would have to experience an illness of truly life-changing proportions; a terminal illness. I have noticed in my work with clients suffering from this kind of problem that the ones who survive are the ones who were prepared to change their whole life; to change their diet, their job, their relationships, their way of thinking and so forth, right down almost to the smallest details. As I mentioned earlier, the power of the mind is such that it is able to hold many conflicting thoughts and beliefs as well as being able to struggle with many of life's difficulties before finally crashing. Sadly, from a soul point of view, the length of time taken for a person to come to this realization is often too long, and through its ability to interact with the pattern body or etheric body it will create a situation whereby some life-threatening disease is going to manifest, thereby giving the person a very powerful signal to re-evaluate their life.

It is the superconscious mind through the etheric body that defines the pattern of flow of all the other frequencies of life energy in the body. The superconscious mind energy is a higher octave of energy again than either the chakra system or the umbilical spiral. It probably functions in a somewhat similar way to the magnetic bottles that were developed by modern atomic physicists to contain plasma, a highly energized form of matter that exists in the heart of the sun. It is the etheric or pattern body; in effect one very high intensity energy field defining the shape of another highly energized field. There has been some confusion concerning the meaning of the word 'etheric body' since it was first used by the theosophists at the end of the last century. It is not related to the throat or ether chakra. It is the phrase they used to express the idea that for anything to flow in a certain pattern it must first have something through which to flow, and secondly the actual shape of the conducting medium would define the pattern of that flow. For example, if you want water to flow in a zig-zag pattern you simply dig a zig-zag shaped ditch and then channel some water in to it.

The boundary of the etheric body is the same as the boundary of the health or physical aura which very definitely follows the contour of the physical body, which is why they called it the etheric body and sometimes the etheric double. They also used the term 'etheric energy' as their generic name for all the different frequencies of life energy that flow within the etheric body. The overall shape of all the different frequencies of life energy was called the aura. Over the last twenty years, as the concept of life energy and energy balancing has spread, many older texts have been re-issued and people who have read them have ascribed their own interpretation to the archaic and scientifically outdated concepts contained within them. These same people have subsequently written books on healing and used these terms with different meanings, adding to the general confusion. I have no doubt that Dr. Stone studied all of the early theosophical texts by Leadbeater et al. My study of the places in his writings where he uses these phrases leads me to believe he did not always use them in their original meaning. This can be very confusing, particularly if you are familiar with the original usage and meaning of the terms.

I have over the last few decades explored a pattern of energy in the human body that I feel is intimately linked to the superconscious mind. A pattern of energy not mapped in Dr. Stone's pioneering work. I have also discovered a number of ways of working with this pattern, but it is not within the scope of this book to explore this area in any further detail.

7. Energy Balancing Techniques

Ear Treatments

The ears are located in the fire oval of the head. They are associated with the ether element, as the sense function associated with ether is hearing. Dr. Stone spoke of the relationship of the ear canal to the head as being the same as that of the umbilicus to the body as a whole. This suggests the possibility of treating any disturbance in the head by polarizing it to the ears and it is also possible to polarize the ear to any other part of the body. He considered the ear canal as the positive pole of the centre of gravity of the body due to the function of the semicircular canals.

The diagnostic areas as represented in the ear are: the upper ear relates to the area above the diaphragm, the middle ear relates to the abdominal area, and the ear lobe relates to the pelvis. Dr. Stone saw the ear lobe as a significant factor in ascertaining the level of vitality a person possessed. Large, plump earlobes indicated a good level of vitality and thus the client would react favourably to any treatment and recover quickly. (Fig.11a, p. 81) Any of these areas on the ear that show redness or discolouration are diagnostic indicators of a disturbance in the organs in that location.

The following treatments release tension in the ear canal and temporomandibular joint (TMJ). They also release the hips through the principle of correspondence. Working the ears can be beneficial in relation to hearing loss and can help with tinnitus, although it is also useful to release the jaw and temporal bones more specifically in these cases.

The client can hum at different pitches whilst the ears are being worked to help clear energy blocks internally with vibration. Working the ear canals is the key to releasing the cranial bones because of the influence they have on the sphenoid bone.

Dr. Stone recommended 4 specific directions for the application of gentle force when working the ears. However, I have found that thinking of the centre of the ear as the hub of a bicycle wheel, with the spokes of the wheel as representing all the different possible lines of force, works well. Thus, it can be beneficial to apply pressure to many lines of force paying particular attention to those that are painful or restricted.

As the earth current line flows around the ear any disturbance in this energy flow can have a negative impact on the function of the ears and so in some cases this current line should be also be released as part of any ear treatment.

Technique 1

Client is on their back

1. Stand at the client's head.
2. Place the earth fingers in the ear canals, keeping the fingers relaxed and open (Fig. 6).
3. Test for tenderness in the ear canal by gently pulling (or pushing) in the directions of force as described in the text on the previous page (Fig. 7).
4. Once you have found a sore line of force, stimulate the ears alternately by applying a gentle pressure in the same direction through the earth fingers (a wiggling movement), until the tenderness has gone.
5. Release all other lines of force that are sore.

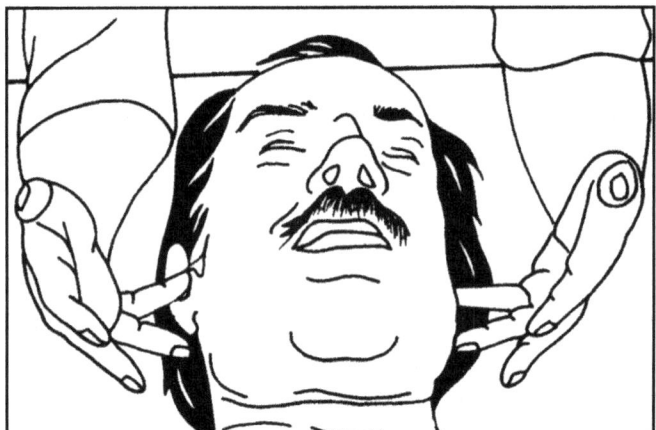

Fig. 6

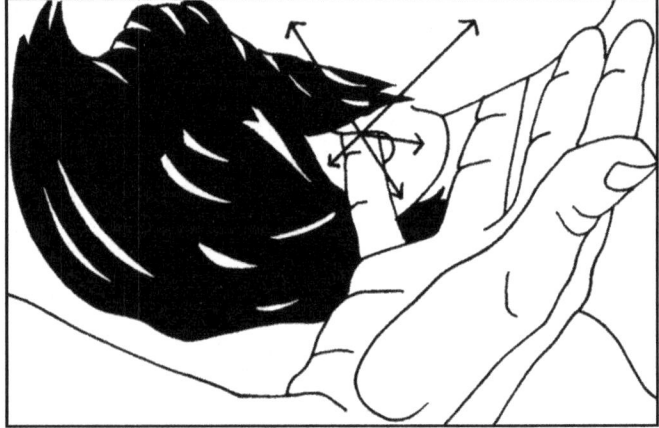

Fig. 7

Technique 2

Client is on their back

1. Stand at the client's head.
2. Place the tip of your air fingers into the ear canal (Fig. 8).
3. Grip the tragus (the small lobe) of each ear between your air fingers and thumbs (Fig. 9).
4. Stimulate each tragus by firmly stretching and rotating it in different directions for about 1 minute. Hold and feel for the energy.

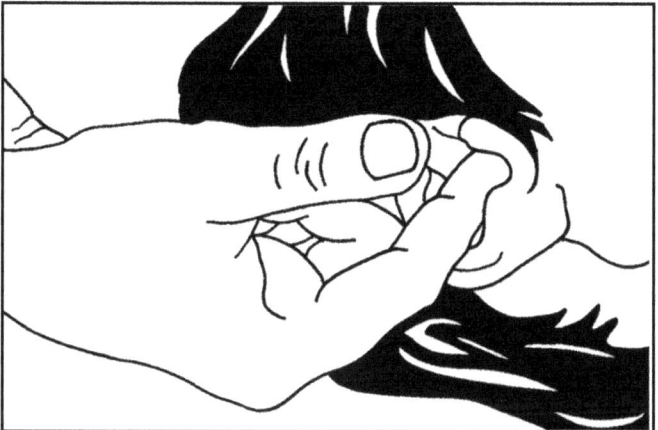

Fig. 8

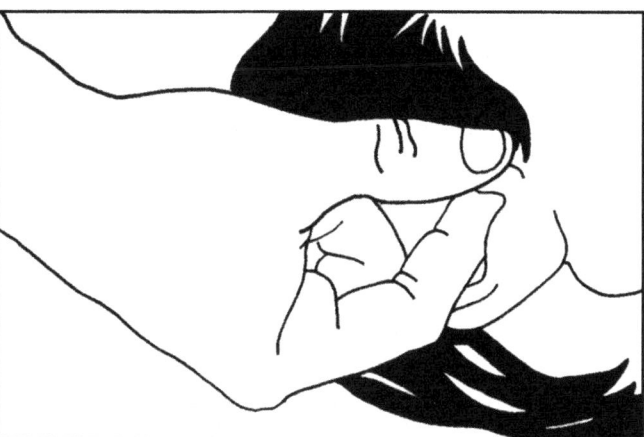

Fig. 9

Technique 3

Client is on their back

1. Stand at the client's head.
2. Place your thumbs in the ears (Fig. 10).
3. Using the fingers to grip the outside of the ears and using the thumbs as a fulcrum, stretch and pull the ear over the thumbs for about 1 minute. Hold and feel for energy. Continue working around the whole of the ear (Fig. 11).

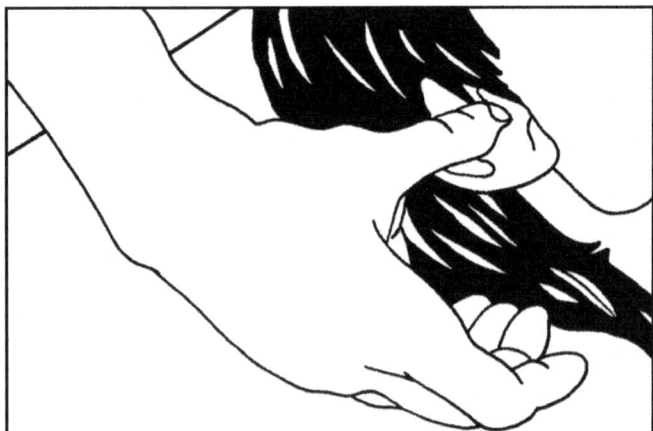

Fig. 10

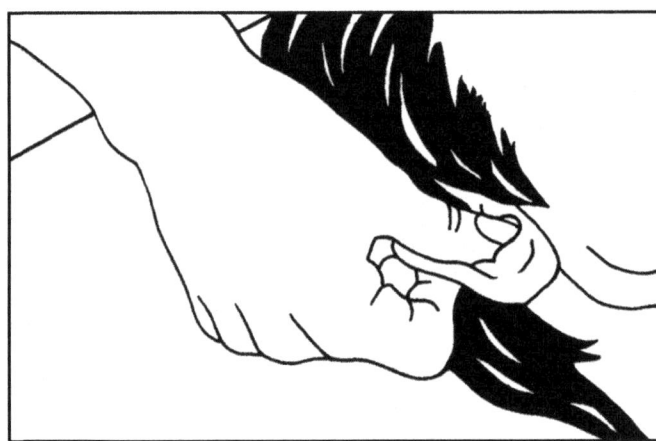

Fig. 11

N.B. The effectiveness of these ear technique can be enhanced by getting the client to hum at a pitch that gives a response in the ears. In fact, any treatment can be enhanced by getting the client to hum at a pitch that resonates with the part of the body being polarized.

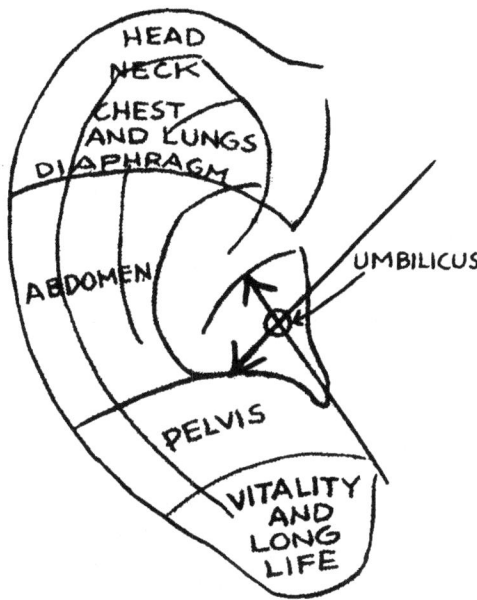

Fig. 11a

Eye/Digestion Treatment

This sensory/motor balance is an excellent release for both the function of the eyes and the digestion as a whole. The occiput is the motor release area for the eyes as well as being a reflex to the abdominal area at the umbilical level. Tension in the occipital base will also tend to create pain in the head and neck. The orbital ridge is a reflex to the diaphragm and is the positive pole of the eyes which are part of the fire astrological triad (eyes, solar plexus, thighs). The manipulation which works the five bi-lateral long line currents at the occiput base and the orbital ridge is useful in cases of headache, digestive disturbance and eye conditions such as conjunctivitis.

Client is on their back

1. Stand at client's head.
2. Place your right fire finger at the left orbital corner near the bridge of the nose and your left air finger on the occipital ridge 1/4 inch to the left of the spine (Fig.12).

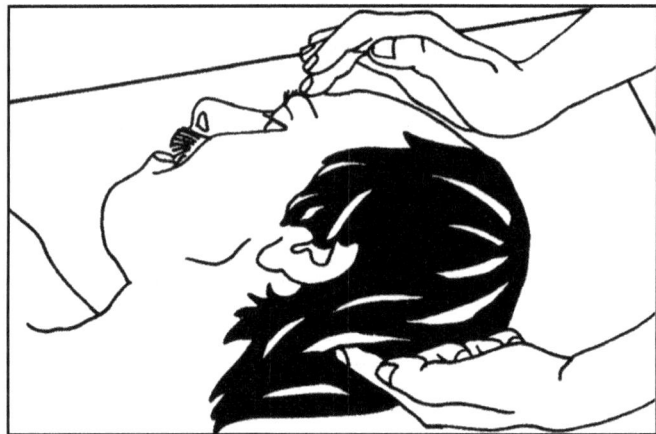

Fig. 12

3. Stimulate alternately for 1 minute.
4. Hold and feel for energy.
5. Continue polarizing all the points along the occipital and orbital ridge working outwards 1/2 inch (1 cm) at a time. Fig. 12 shows the technique at mid–point on the two ridges.
6. Repeat on the right side using the left air finger on the orbital ridge and the right fire finger on the occipital ridge.

N.B. This whole treatment can be done with diagonal contacts.

Cranial Moulding

Cranial moulding is an approach to cranial release that does not rely on working any specific rhythms of cranial energetic pulsations. Instead it just simply seeks to release the cranial sutures and energy in a general way so that the cerebro–spinal impulse is freed. The self regulating nature of the cerebro–spinal system ensures that the energy released comes into balance of its own accord. It releases the fire element oval and the circulation of the prana in the cerebro–spinal fluid. The cranial sutures need only a light touch to free them when fixed, just as a pendulum needs only a light touch to set it in motion.

These cranial moulding techniques can have a profound effect upon the sinuses in the skull. They are not referenced in Dr. Stone's writings as such but they are shown in his book Health Building as contacts upon the skull that one can do whilst squatting.

Client is seated

(The height of the stool on which the client sits should allow their head to be at your chest level)

1. Stand behind the client.
2. Place both hands over the client's ears, fingers pointing towards the top of the head, so that the heel of the palm hooks the mastoid process and the angle of the jaw on each side (Fig. 13).

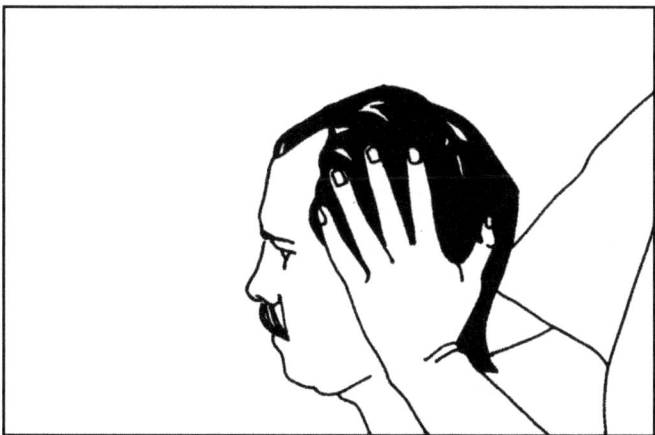

Fig. 13

3. Apply a slight upward and inward lift on the head as if trying to lift it away from the shoulders, at the same time as you are gently squeezing it. Once the head is at full lift apply a gentle vibration through the hands for ten seconds. Relax the lift for ten seconds and repeat this sequence 3 or 4 times.

4. Stand on the client's left side.
5. Place the heel of your left palm so that it is hooked beneath the orbital ridge over the bridge of the nose, and the heel of your right palm hooks the central portion of the occipital ridge (Fig. 14).

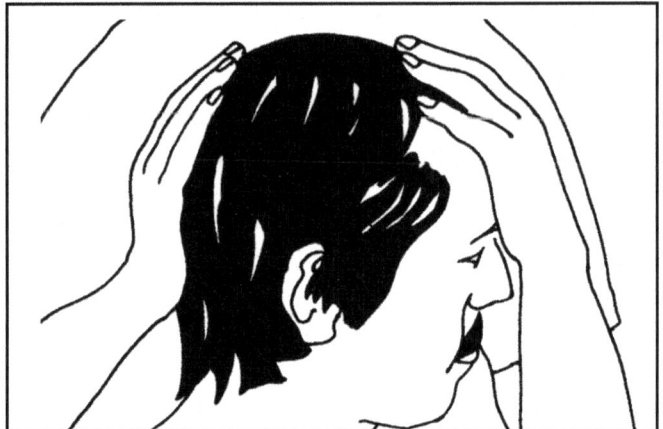

Fig. 14

6. Lift, squeeze and vibrate as in step 3. Repeat 3 or 4 times, resting between each lift.
7. Stay on the client's left side.
8. Place your left hand so that the heel of the palm hooks beneath the left outer edge of the orbital ridge, and the heel of your right palm hooks beneath the right mastoid process (Fig. 15).

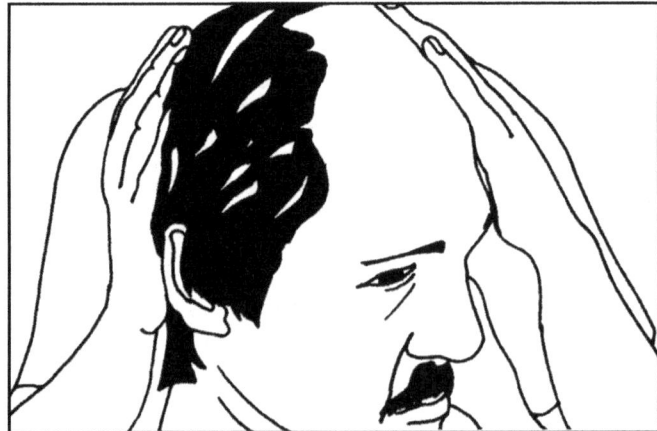

Fig. 15

9. Lift, squeeze and vibrate exactly as in step 6.
10. Stand on the client's right side. Repeat steps 8 and 9. This time the contacts are on the right outer orbital ridge and left mastoid process.

11. Stand behind the client.
12. Place the heels of the palms over the temples with the fingers overlapping on the forehead (Fig. 16).

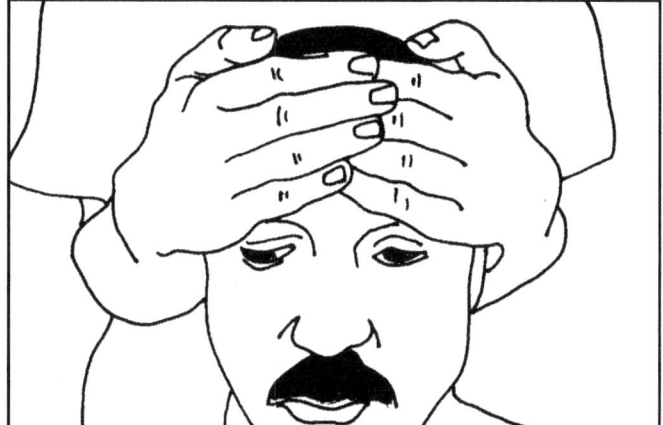

Fig. 16

13. Apply a gentle squeezing movement to the client's temples, alternately increasing and decreasing the pressure every few seconds for about 1 minute.
14. Ask the client to lie down on the table and stand on their right side.
15. Place your right thumb over their left cheek bone and allow the palm to mould to the face, and the heel of your left palm over their forehead just above the right eye (Fig. 17).

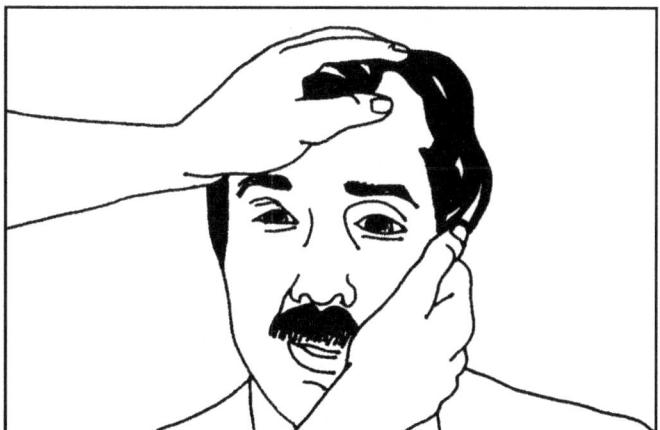

Fig. 17

16. Apply a slight downward and outward stretch and then vibrate the cheek contact for about 30 seconds.
17. Repeat on the opposite side from right cheek to left forehead.

Cranial Relationships

Fig. 18 shows how the skull, symbolizing the creative mind patterns, steps down through the various oval fields of the body. It is a representation of consciousness pervading the body and setting up harmonic relationships in the process. It shows how the energy of the central nervous system innervates the body. The three poles of the central nervous system are the cranium as the positive pole, the shoulder area as the neutral pole and the pelvis as the negative pole.

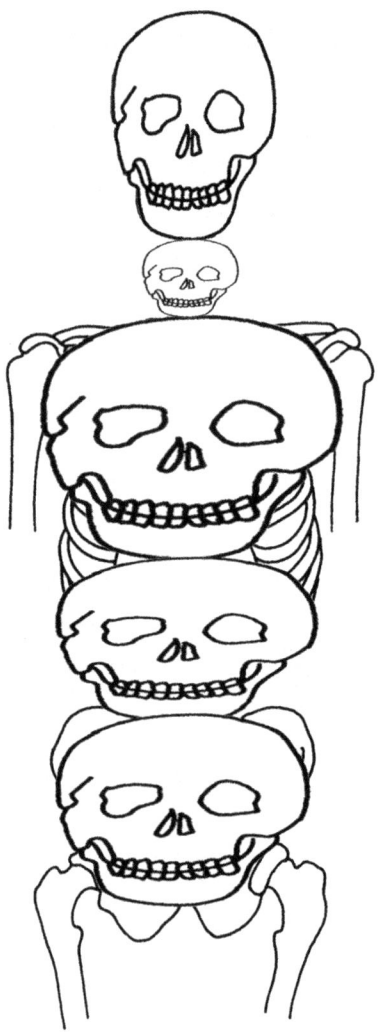

Fig. 18

The figure shows various relationships between the head and neck, head and chest, head and abdomen and head and pelvis. It also gives a basic proportional relationship between all of the five oval fields in the body. For example the pupil of the eye, which lies on the air current line, in approximately the centre of the fire oval, has four other nodal points that have powerful reflex relationships to it, the points being on the air current line approximately in the middle of each of the other four oval fields.

These points are shown in Fig. 19. Therefore, an excellent treatment for the eyes is to place the fingertips over the eye to be treated and polarize it, using alternate stimulation, to each of the other four nodal points in turn.

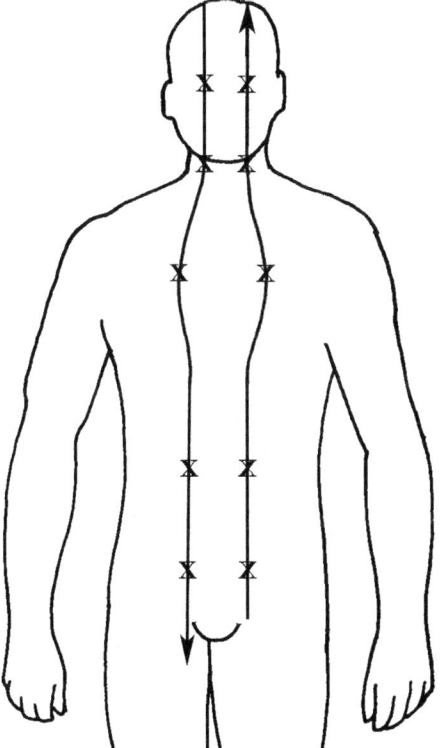

Fig. 19

Cranial/Pelvic Balance

This cranial-pelvic session is a balancing of the central nervous system at its positive pole in the cranium and its negative pole in the pelvis. In this session we are connecting reflex areas on the head to corresponding areas on the pelvis. It is effective in all conditions of the head or pelvis and for mental-emotional problems as it balances the conscious mind in its action as thinking in the head with the unconscious mind and its expression in the pelvis. It is a balancing of the fire and water elements, the interlaced triangles (or 6-pointed star pattern) and is an excellent way to finish any Polarity treatment.

Client is on their back

1. Stand on the client's right side.
2. Place your left hand obliquely along the line of the jaw, and the fingers of your right hand on the right side of the symbiosis pubis (Fig. 20).

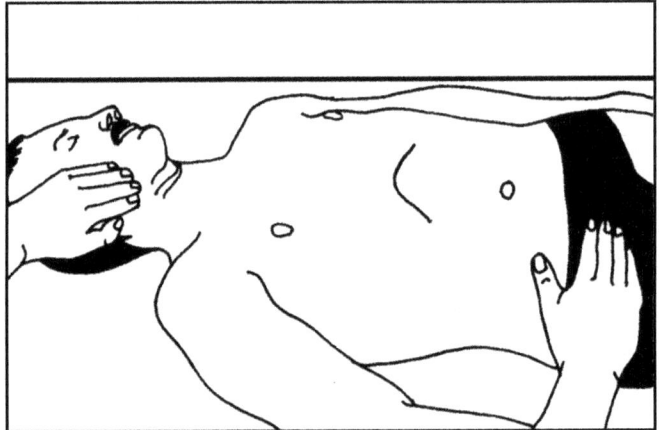

Fig. 20

3. Feel for the energy in the pelvis and once you have a sense of its rhythm or vibration, rock the jaw to the same rhythm taking about 2 minutes altogether.
4. Repeat on the other side of the body
5. Stay on the client's left side.
6. Place your right thumb over the maxilla just to the left side of the nose, with the

fingers spread out on the side of the head, and your left hand cups the right iliac crest (Fig. 21).

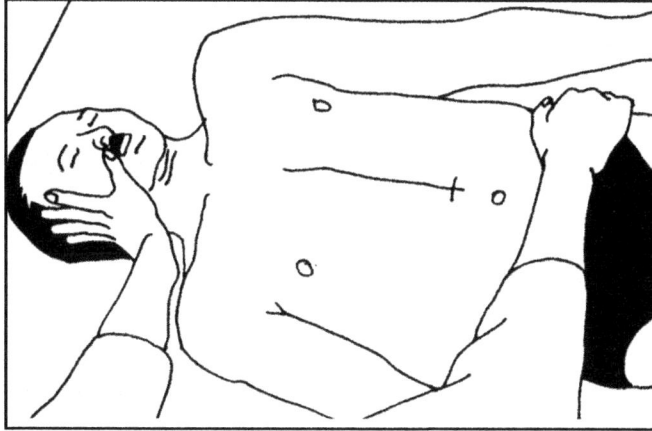

Fig. 21

7. Stimulate by rocking the iliac crest for 1–2 minutes. Hold and feel for the energy.
8. Repeat on the other side of the body .
9. Come back to the client's right side.
10. Place the left hand over the forehead and the right hand between the iliac crests (Fig. 22).

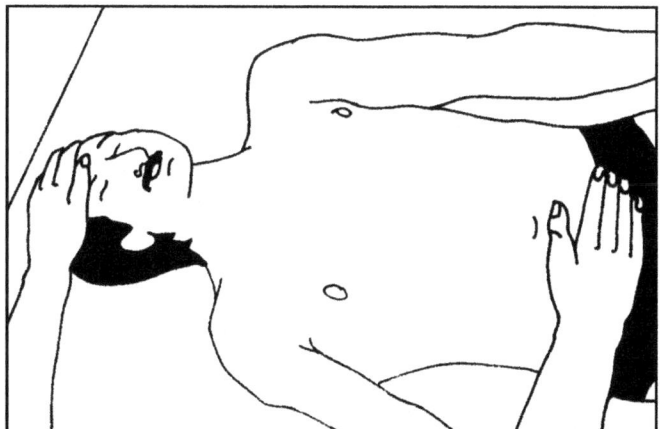

Fig. 22

11. Rock the pelvic contact very softly, the range of movement is no more than 1/4 inch, for 1–2 minutes. Hold and feel for energy.

12. Move the left hand slowly from the forehead and gently grip the bridge of the nose between the thumb and air finger. Peel the right hand slowly off the pelvis until you just have the outer edge of the palm left in contact (Fig. 23).

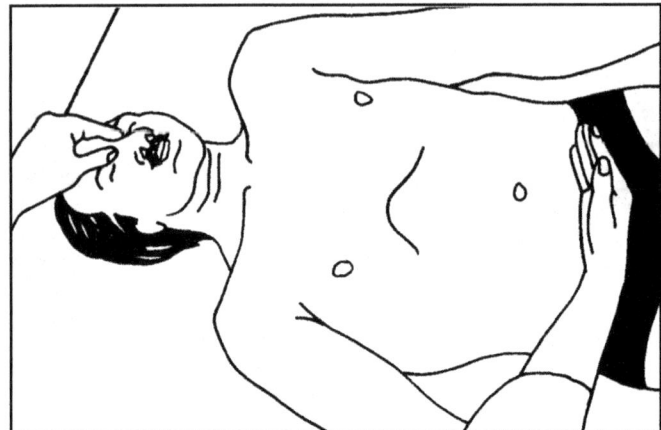

Fig. 23

13. Stimulate the pelvis through the edge of the right palm as in step 11.
14. Take the hands slowly off the body when finished.

The cranial / pelvic relationships upon which this treatment is based is set out below and is derived from Fig. 18 p. 86.

Jaw	Symphysis pubis
Parietal bones	Ilium
Maxilla	Inguinal ligament
Frontal bone	Lower abdomen
Nasal bone	Mid–point in pelvic oval

Heart Therapy

Dr. Stone outlined three primary reasons for heart problems. The first he describes as emotional problems to do with the head and the heart and the lack of communication between the two. The second has more to do with poor digestion and eating foods rich in fats that impair the blood flow through the arteries and raise blood pressure. Poor digestion is often the cause of a build up of gas in the stomach and colon which can also put excess pressure on the heart causing it to work too hard against the resistance. The third cause has more to do with structural problems of the heart itself, such as valve malfunction, or a difficulty in the electrical impulses which keep it beating regularly. Of course, in practice, a heart problem could be caused by any one or all three of these conditions.

The nature of a specific of a heart problem can be ascertained by checking for tenderness between the tendon interspaces of the left hand and foot as well as checking for any distortions of the air, fire and water fingers. The areas of most tenderness in a specific reflex area(s) is your guide and you then treat accordingly. If in doubt treat the reflexes between the thumb/big toe and the air finger/toe as this is the most direct reflex to the area of the chest and heart. Remember that when treating a client with a heart condition it may be very uncomfortable for them to lie flat as breathing can be difficult in this position, so treat them in a sitting or supported position.

Fig. 24 overleaf shows the location of the tendon interspaces marked as areas 1, 2, 3 and 4. These particular areas are horizontal reflex areas and are useful both as diagnostic indicators and areas for polarization.

The areas correspond to the following organs.

1	Neck	Brachial Plexus	impulse to liver and diaphragm
2	Diaphragm	Lungs	brachial plexus (respiratory organs)
3.	Kidneys	duodenum	jejunum (digestive organs)
4.	Prostate	uterus	rectum (generative organs)

N.B. These areas and correspondences are the same on both left and right hands and feet.

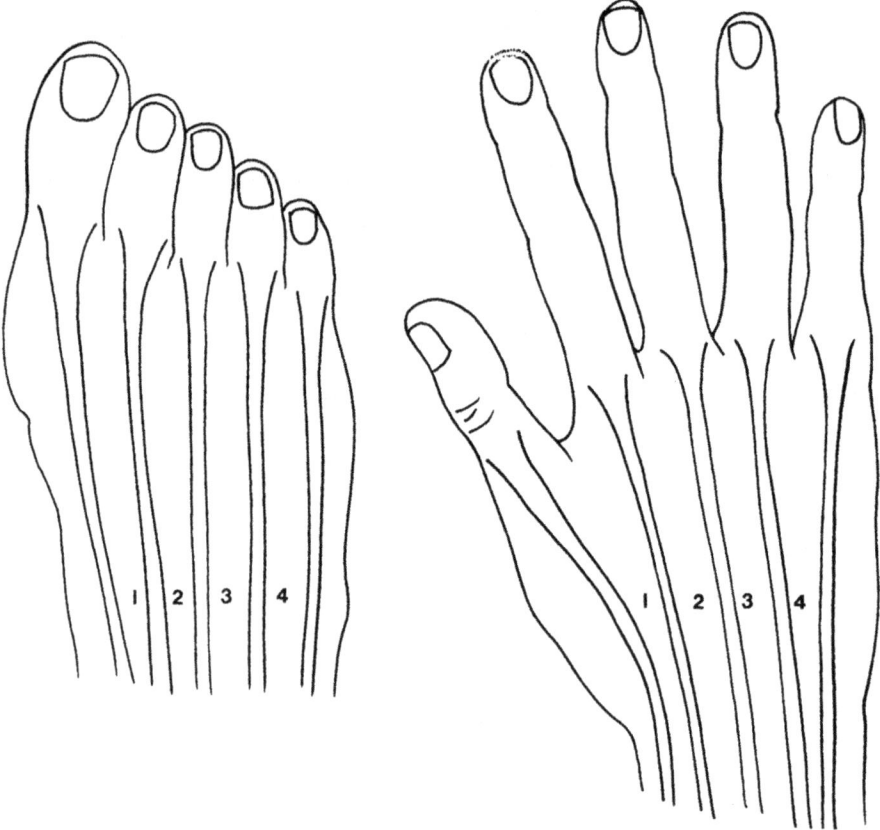

Fig. 24

For heart problems check the left hand, the particular joint to check of the air, fire and water fingers is the first joint in each. The air finger is the true polarity reflex to the heart. When it is sore, in cases of heart trouble, then the air element is being over stressed and rest from mental, emotional strain is most important. It is indicative of a hypertension as the main factor. Soreness of tendon interspace 1 is also indicative of this kind of problem being the neck area, which is the link between the head and the heart.

When the first joint of the fire finger or tendon interspace 2 is sore, then it is the warmth in the circulation that is in trouble due to poor digestion and the probable accumulation of fatty deposits in the arteries and veins. When the first joint of the water finger and tendon interspace 3 is sore, then it is the watery matrix of the heart structure and the impulse for it to pump that are in trouble.

The same relationships are true of the air, fire and water toes and tendon interspaces of the right foot. Remember the feet show chronic energy blocks and the hands acute energy blocks.

Client is on their back

1. Stand at the client's feet.
2. Polarize the first joints of the air, fire and water toes on both feet. Begin polarizing both air toes simultaneously by gently pulling and squeezing them for 1 minute or until any tenderness has gone. continue with the fire and water toes in the same way.
3. Polarize the tendon interspaces 1, 2 and 3 on both feet.Grip each foot between your thumb and fingers so that the thumb is underneath the foot and the fingers lie in the tendon interspace. Begin with tendon interspace 1 (Fig. 25).

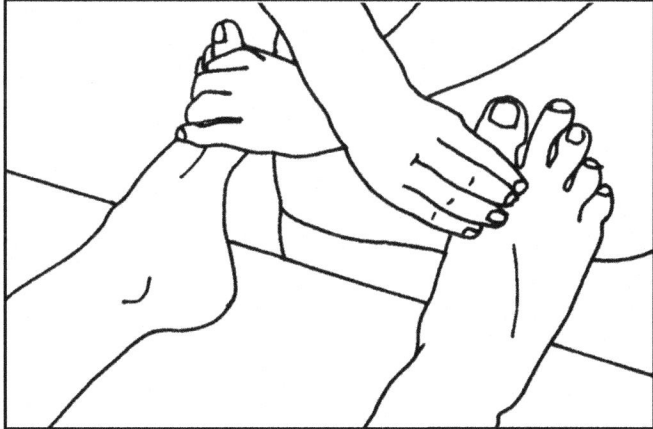

Fig. 25

4. Stimulate by rhythmically squeezing the sore areas for 1 minute or until the tenderness disappears It is sometimes easier to do this technique with the arms crossed.
5. Polarize the fingers and tendon interspaces in the hands in the same way. See Fig. 26 overleaf for the tendon interspace grip on the hands.

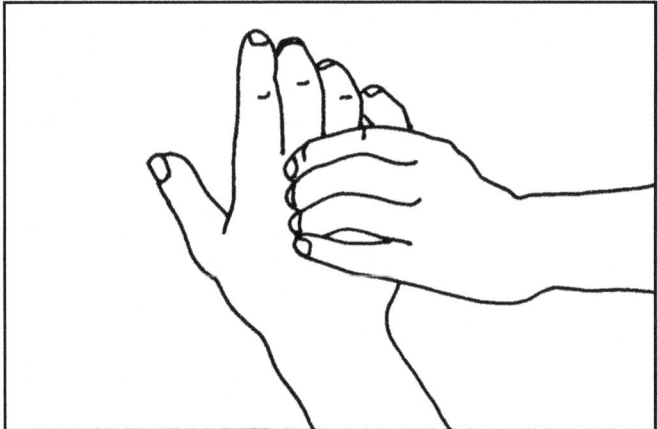

Fig. 26

6. Release the brachial plexus on both sides.
7. Stand on the client's right side.
8. Place your right thumb at the tip of the sternum just beneath the xiphoid process, and the left hand grips the right shoulder with the thumb beneath the clavicle (Fig. 27).

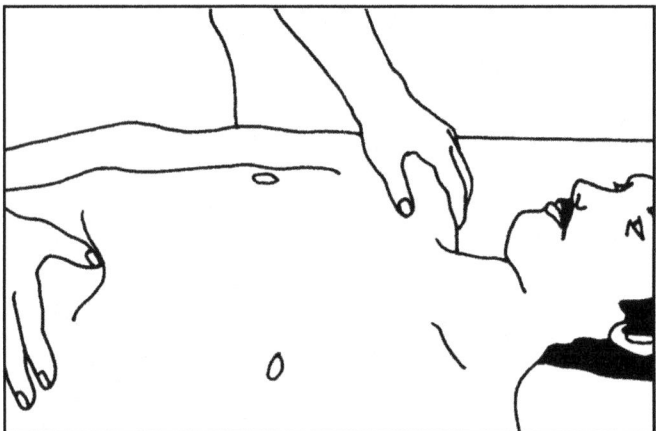

Fig. 27

9. Rhythmically squeeze the muscles over the right shoulder and alternate this with a directional contact of the thumb up under the ribs towards the right shoulder. Work along the line of the right lower ribs, releasing any tender areas. In some cases, due to the amount of tension, the little finger has to be used instead of the thumb.
10. Staying on the same side of the client's body, reach across to the left shoulder with your left hand and free any tender area along the left lower ribs, using the same techniques as in Step 8.

Steps 5–9 are specifically aimed at releasing any tension or spasticity in the diaphragm. The diaphragm is the most important muscle in relation to heart function, and its balanced functioning is a vital factor to achieve in any heart therapy. Details on the specifics of releasing the brachial plexus are in the book *Polarity Therapy - Healing with Life Energy.*[1]

11. Still on the right side of the client's body, place your right thumb once more at the xiphoid process, pointing upwards. To stimulate the heart function the left thumb is placed over the third eye, with the fingers on the section of the line of cardiac stability that is above the left ear (Fig. 28). The cardiac stability is shown in Fig. 28a.

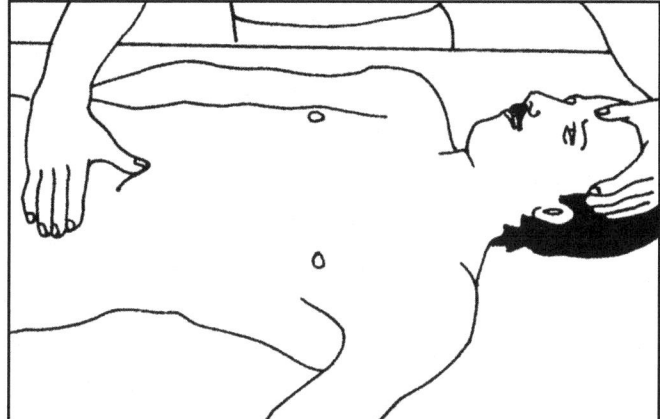

Fig. 28

12. Stimulate the cardiac stability with a gentle movement of the left fingers, as you hold the right thumb contact steady for about 1 minute.

13. To relax the heart function the left hand is laid along the line of the left side of the jaw, and the thumb of the right hand at the xiphoid process is directed towards the jaw contact (Fig. 29 overleaf).

14. There is no stimulation in this technique. It is a satvic hold.

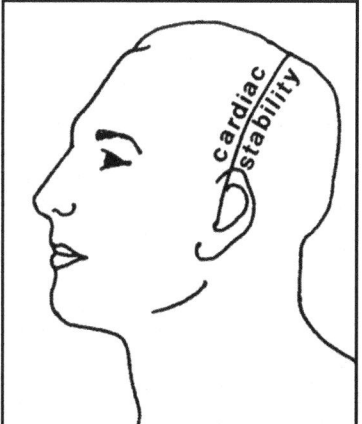

Fig. 28a

1. by Alan Siegel M.S. N.D. and Phil Young, Published by Masterworks International, 2006

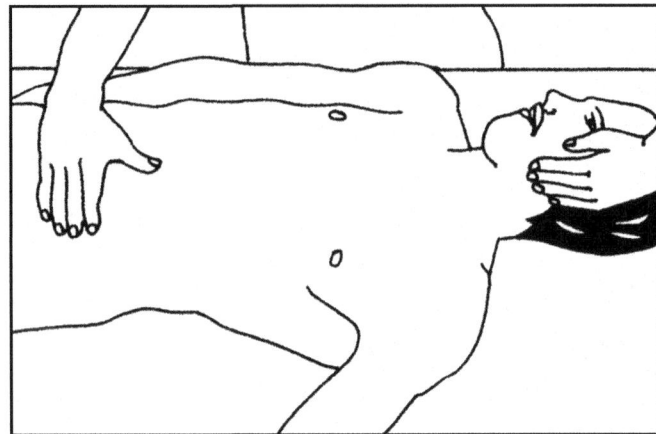

Fig. 29

N.B. The cardiac stability (Fig. 28a, previous page) is a cranial control reflex for heart function. It runs along the line of the left side of the jaw, through the ear, and then parallels the line of the frontal! parietal bone sutures at about the middle of the parietal bone. The upper section of the line is the contact area for tonifying heart action, the lower section for sedating it. Tonify or sedate the heart according to the client's needs.

Contacts With and Against Surface Current Flow

These techniques are used for releasing the fascia and either stimulating or relaxing the long line currents of the body as well as releasing local energy blocks anywhere on the body. One or two hands may be used when applying the technique, whichever gives the best response. The main energetic effect of these techniques is created by the directional impulse behind them, not on the actual polarity of your contacts. All these techniques are done using the whole body to give momentum to the technique. The nature of the contacts is a low amplitude pulse. It is important to maintain an overall relaxation throughout the whole body when applying these techniques.

Contacts that are applied with the current flow are soothing in their effect, and contacts against the current flow are stimulating. Contacts with the current flow are used where there is heat, pain and inflammation, and contacts against current flow are used when there is muscular spasm, paralysis or excess tension. In all the techniques you should vary the angle of application until you get the best response. This type of treatment can be given at the beginning of a session to generally stimulate or sedate the energy and can be used on the front of the body at the start of a structural session to release anterior energy blocks and unlock sensory holding.

Technique 1

Client is on their front

1. Stand on the client's left side.
2. Place your left palm on the upper back at a 45 degree angle (Fig. 30).

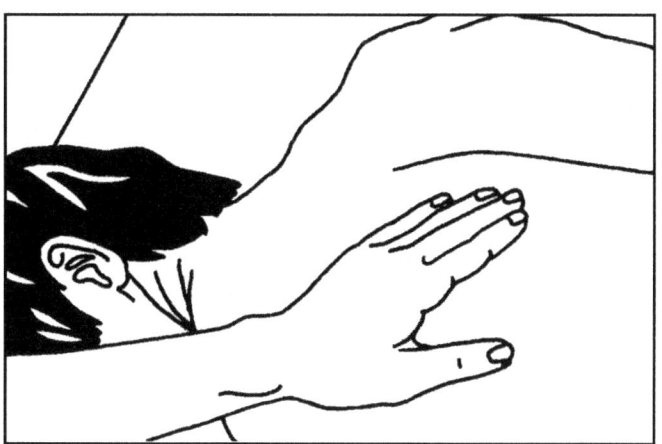

Fig. 30

3. Twist your left hand until the fingers are pointing downwards, whilst maintaining a firm but relaxed contact with the skin, thereby taking up the slack in the underlying tissues (Fig. 31).

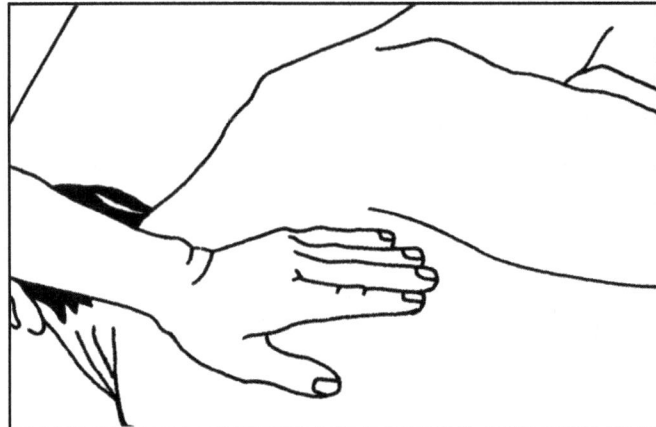

Fig. 31

4. Firm your contact by placing the right hand on top of the left hand (Fig. 32).

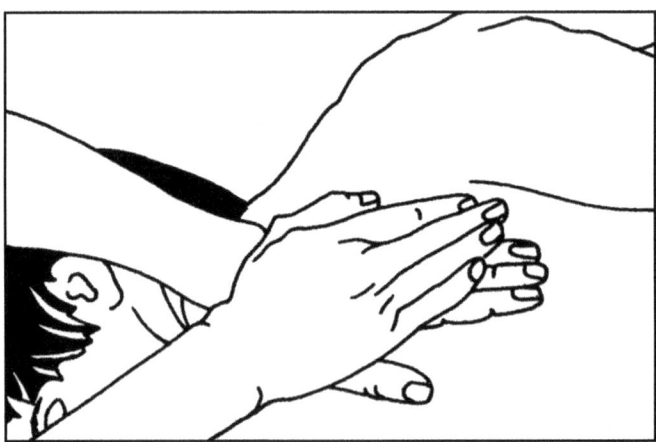

Fig. 32

5. Shifting your weight to the balls of your feet, pulse the client's body by rocking backwards and forwards for 1–2 minutes. Make sure you use your whole body to achieve the pulsing, not just your arms (Fig. 33).

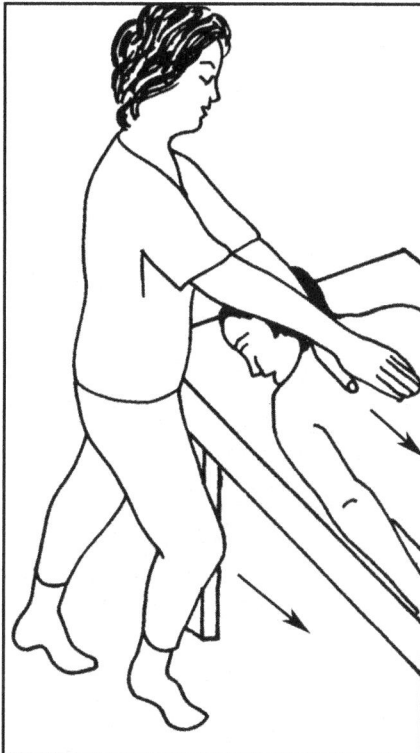

Fig. 33

Technique 2

Client is on their back

1. Stand on the client's right side.
2. Place your left hand over the client's right lower abdomen so that the fingers over the pubic bone are pointing downwards, and your right hand is on the upper thigh with the fingers also pointing downwards (Fig. 34).

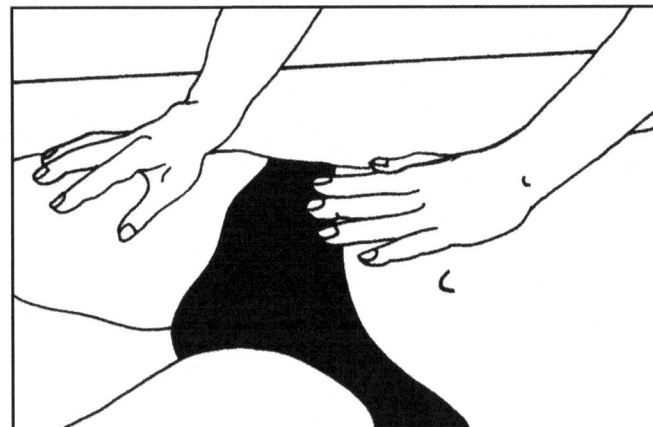

Fig. 34

3. Using your whole body as in step 5 of technique 1, pulse downwards towards the feet for 1–2 minutes. Make sure your hands do not slide over the skin.
4. Stand on the client's left side.
5. Place your left hand on the client's left upper thigh, fingers pointing upwards, and your right hand on the abdomen so that the finger tips are pushing gently up underneath the floating ribs on the left side (Fig. 35).
6. As in Step 3 pulse your hands upwards towards the head for 1–2 minutes.

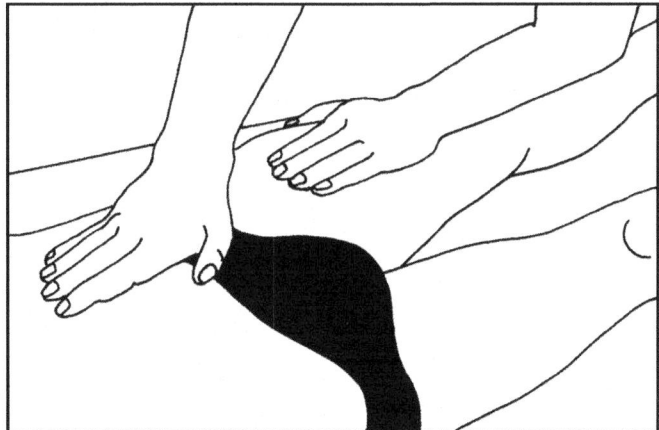

Fig. 35

Technique 3

This particular technique polarizes the spine by creating an opposing stretch in the muscles on either side. It can be done anywhere along the spine where tension, pain or spasm exists.

Client is on their front

1. Stand on the client's left side.
2. Place your left hand over the spine at a 45 degree angle so that the palm is covering the mid-dorsal vertebrae, and place your right palm over the top as a support (Fig. 36).

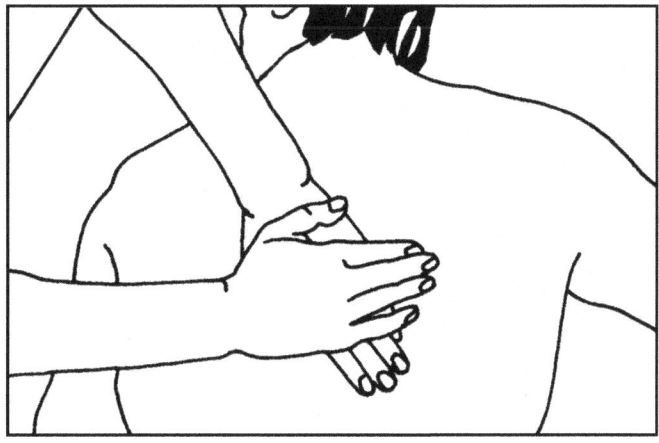

Fig. 36

101

3. Applying firm pressure twist your hands anticlockwise (Fig. 37).

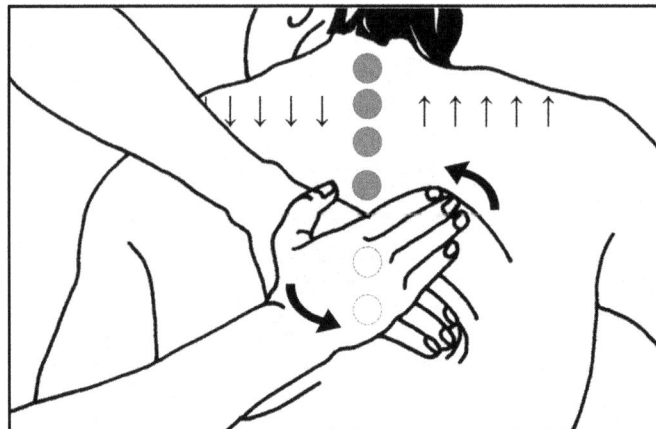

Fig. 37

4. Holding the muscles under tension, pulse your hands upwards towards the head by using a rocking movement of your whole body until the muscles relax. Vibratory impulses may be used instead.
5. Move up and down working all spinal areas required.

N.B. The three techniques above are demonstrated *with* the current flow.

Muscular Drainage by Opposing Forces

(The 'S' Technique)

This technique was recommended by Dr. Stone as one of the simplest and most effective ways of draining a muscle of stagnant material. It is best done against the local current flow as a stimulating contact. As well as being a muscle drainage technique it is also an excellent way to release the fascia. It is a useful technique for releasing muscular and energetic tension either side of the spine prior to doing any kind of vertebral work.

Reddening of the skin indicates energetic stagnation and is a positive response as it shows increased energy and blood flow in the area. The technique can be effectively combined with skin rolling. A toxic response such as headache or feeling of dis-ease may result after draining the musculature. A common response to work on the muscles of the back, where we are releasing accumulated muscle tension, is excessive itching as the energy breaks through the surface restriction and the skin becomes enlivened.

Client is on their front

1. Stand on the client's left side.
2. Place your right thumb on the left side of a tense muscle fibre and your left thumb on the right side. The tensest muscles are often near the spine (Fig. 38).

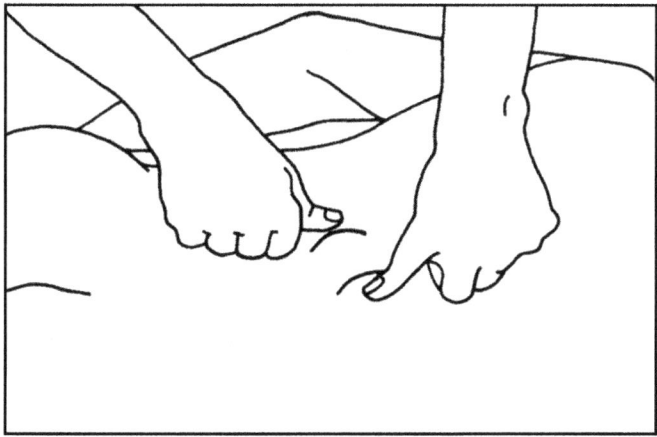

Fig. 38

3. Push your right thumb upwards and your left thumb downwards, making sure that they do not slide, thereby creating an 'S' shaped fold in the tissues (Fig. 39).

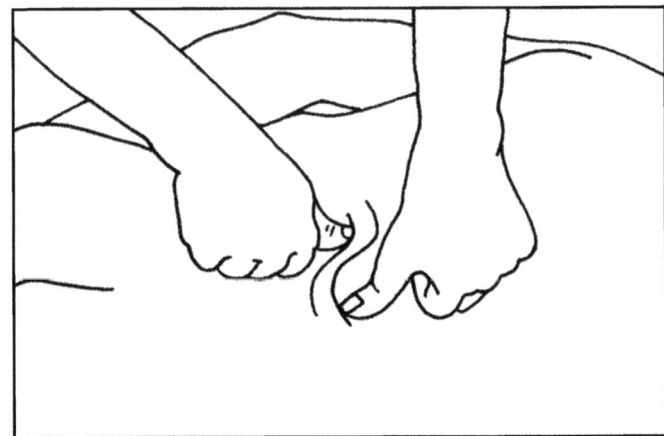

Fig. 39

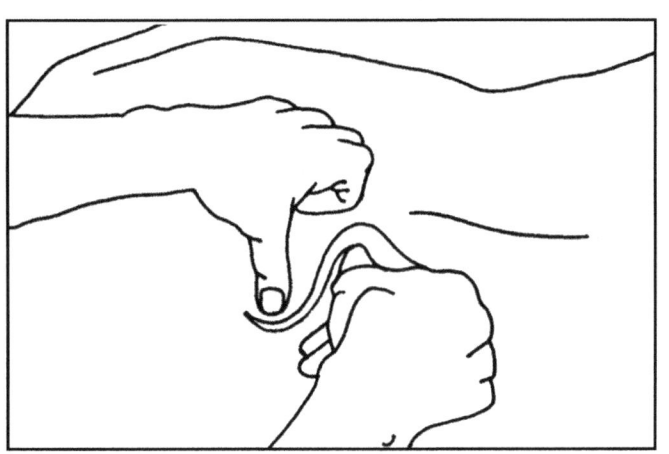

Fig. 40

4. The same basic technique can be done horizontally on the body (Fig. 40). It can also be done using the whole hand (Fig. 41).

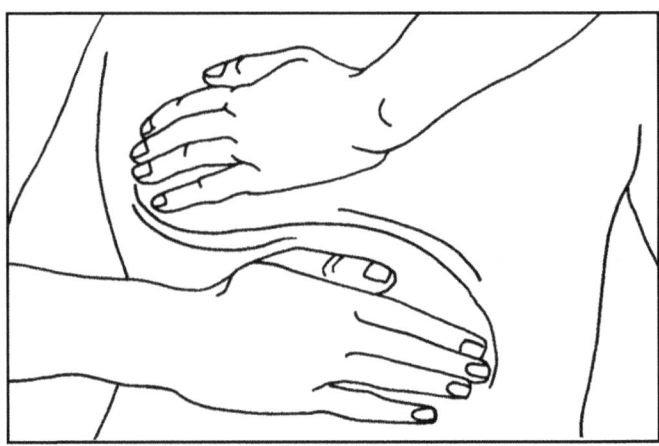

Fig. 41

Digestive Treatment

This is an earth element treatment. It uses part of the astrological triad of the earth element (knees, bowels and neck) as represented by the knees, and the earth element's physical area of function, the abdominal oval field. It also utilises the influence of the 5-pointed star energy pattern by the work over the Poupart's ligament to help clear energy blocks in the digestive organs. Both support for and influences from the five pointed star pattern are carried through the legs and arms. Sometimes this two way influence can give rise to elbow and knee problems which have their roots in the digestive system. Conversely disturbances in the energy around the knees and elbows can cause digestive disturbance. The 5-pointed star influence, which crosses over in the torso, explains why pain in the right knee is often a reflex from the stomach on the opposite side of the body and in the left knee from the liver/gall bladder.

Client is on their back.

1. Stand on the client's left side.
2. Place your left hand over the left knee and the fingertips of your right hand over the Poupart's ligament on the left side (Fig. 42).

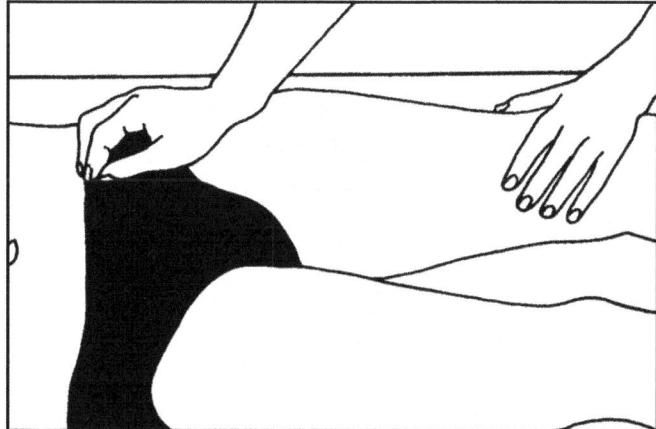

Fig. 42

3. Stimulate alternately by rocking the knee gently and working your fingers gently down in to the pelvis, then up towards the opposite shoulder with a scooping movement for 1–2 minutes. Hold and feel for the energy.

4. Move your left hand to the Poupart's ligament on the left side and your right hand to the liver area on the opposite side of the body. The fingertips of the right hand can be placed just up underneath the floating ribs on the right side if required (Fig. 43).

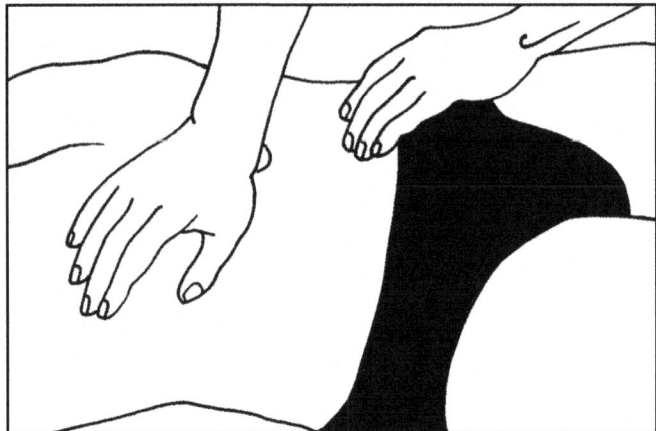

Fig. 43

5. Stimulate the Poupart's ligament as in step 3, and alternate it with a gentle rocking of the liver area up towards the right shoulder alternately for 1–2 minutes. Hold and feel for the energy.
6. Move your left hand back to the left knee, the right stays on the liver area (Fig. 44).

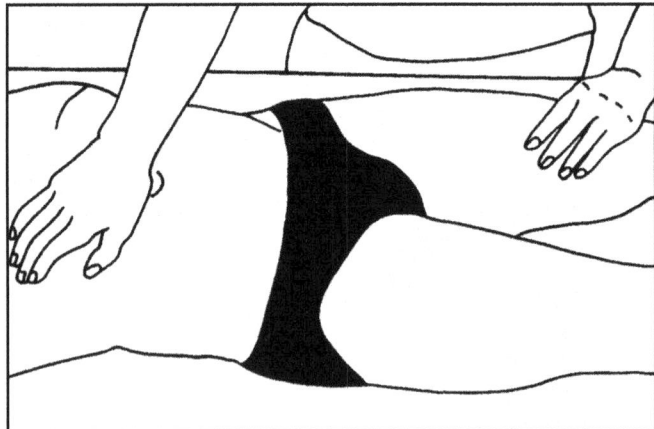

Fig. 44

7. Stimulate alternately by rocking the knee and the liver area for 1–2 minutes. Hold and feel for the energy.
8. Repeat manipulations 1–7 on the client's right side. Remember to cross over to the stomach.

Balancing by Contour

Balancing by Contour is the name given by Dr. Stone to treating blocked areas in the body on the basis of the hermetic principle of correspondence. I also use the term 'symmetry of form' as an alternative title for this kind of balancing work. In essence, it means that those areas of the body that have similar contour or shape have a definite energetic relationship to each other. I will explore the concept in more detail in the chapter on structural balancing. The sore spots in a particular area can be released by polarizing them to points in other areas of similar shape. Fig. 45 shows dotted areas as contact points in the pelvic girdle below relating to similar points in the shoulder girdle above. As an example the curved, rounded area over the shoulders has a correspondence to the rounded area of the buttocks.

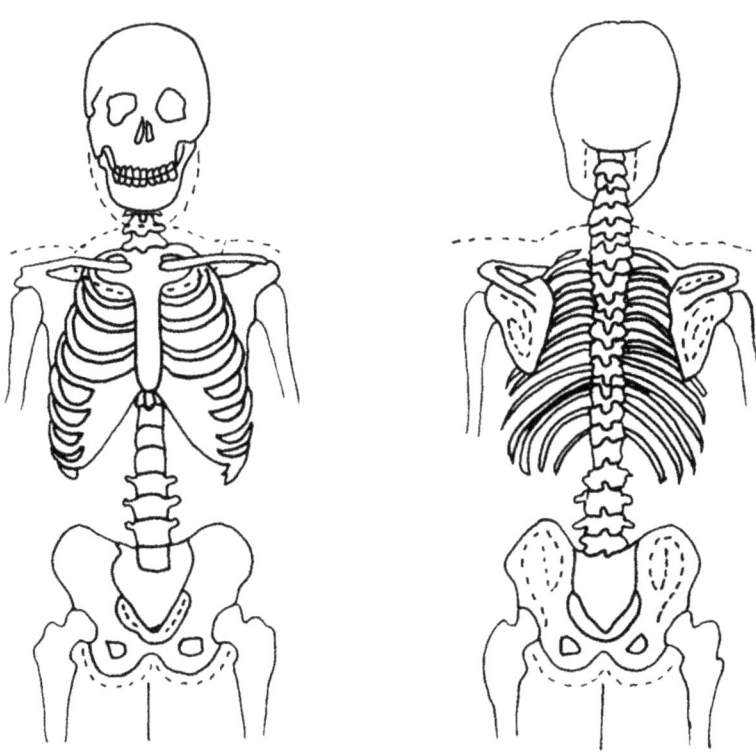

Fig. 45

From an elemental point of view, working the buttocks and shoulders is a balancing of the air and water elements, and releasing the strain in these areas results in a definite improvement in the quality of movement. There is also a strong effect on the structure of the body as the anti-gravity muscles of the buttocks and back are being influenced. Work on the buttocks and scapula also activates the sympathetic nervous system. Highly stressed, sympathetic dominant types frequently have excessive tension in these areas and can benefit enormously from their release. The treatment can also be used as a balancing of the parasympathetic nervous system specifically when the contacts shift to the upper part of the upper gluteal muscles which are supplied by the sacral parasympathetic nerves and their contour balancing area in the upper back along the top line of the shoulders and lower neck which are supplied by the vagus and the spinal accessory nerves, which are themselves part of the parasympathetic nervous system.

Client is on their front

1. Stand on the client's left side.
2. Using your right thumb find the sorest spot over the left buttock, and with your left thumb the sorest spot over the left scapula.
3. Holding the sore spot over the scapula with your left thumb, stimulate the sore area on the buttock with your right. Try using different directions of gentle force on the buttock contact until the tenderness in both areas is gone. You may also use alternate stimulation if you wish (Fig. 46).

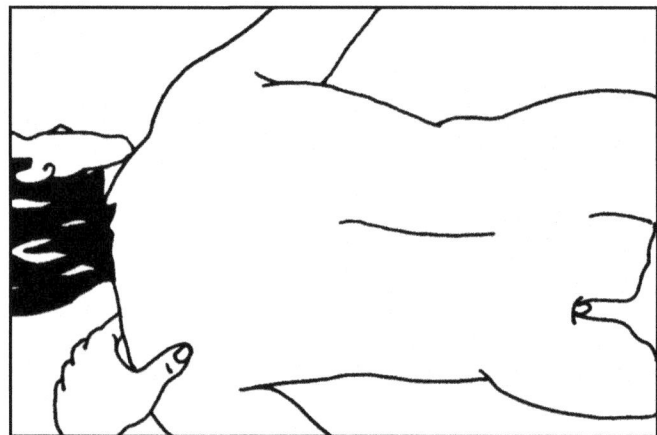

Fig. 46

4. Repeat on the client's right side.
5. In some cases the stress and strain may cross diagonally to the other side of the body,

in which case the contacts are from buttock to opposite shoulder. Releasing the buttock muscles to the scapula on the opposite side is an excellent way of freeing the diaphragm. Use the same procedure as in steps 2–4 but making diagonal contacts (Fig. 47).

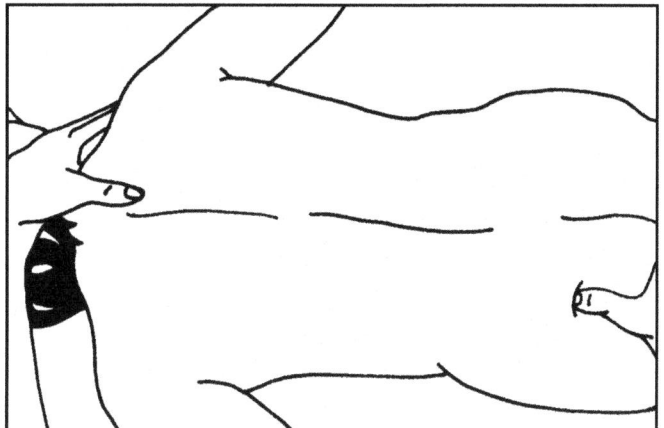

Fig. 47

Breast Treatment

This treatment, which is very useful in treating lumps and stagnation in the breasts is, in essence, a balancing of the posterior motor poles of the water element. The scapula area is the motor pole of the breasts, the buttocks provide the push (motor action) to the genitals, and the calves provide the motive power to the feet. The actual areas for treatment are shown in Fig. 48.

This treatment also uses the idea of blancing by contour. In this case the rounded area of the calf muscles is also included along with the rounded buttocks and back of the shoulders. Stagnation in the motor aspect of the water energy can cause problems in all anterior watery areas. This treatment is recommended for lumpy, painful and swollen tissue in the breasts (specific lumps should always be checked out by a medical doctor). It encourages the free flow of the water element throughout the body. It can also be effective in cases where there is a general acute sensitivity all over the body indicating an problem with the water element.

Client is on their front

1. Stand on the client's left side.
2. Place the left hand palm down over the left buttock, and the right hand palm down over the calf area, fingers pointing towards the head. The contact areas are as shaded in Fig. 48.
3. Stimulate by simultaneously pulsing both contacts in a headward direction for 1–2 minutes.
4. Move the left palm up to the left scapula and the right palm to the left buttock.
5. Stimulate as in step 3.
6. Leave the left palm on the scapula and move the right palm back down to the calf area. Depending on the client, this may be a long stretch, you may need to bend the client's leg, supporting it in the crook of your arm with your palm on the calf muscle.
7. Stimulate as in step 3.
8. Repeat on the right side of the client's body.

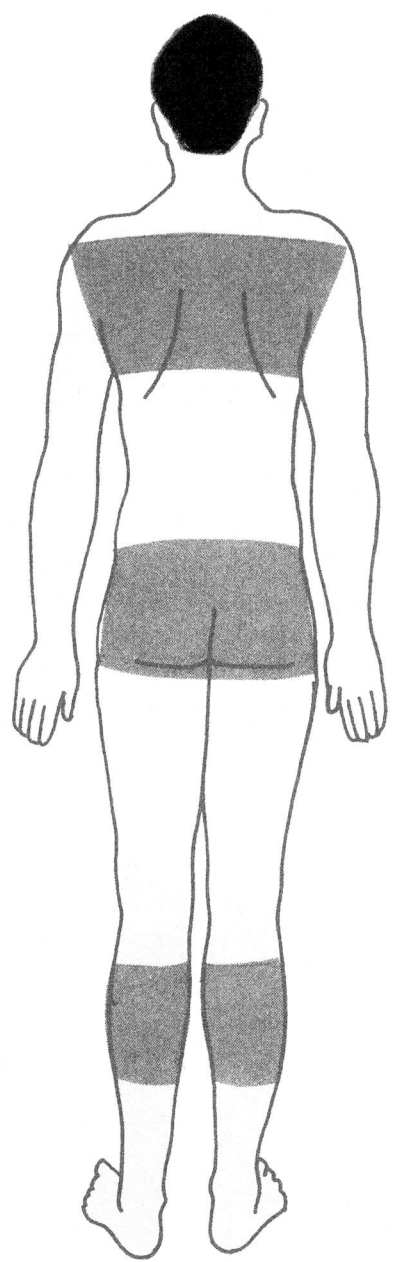

Fig. 48

Seated Release of Neck and Dorsal Vertebrae

This is one of Dr. Stone's *country-side techniques*, used when you do not have access to a table and where the manipulation is performed with the client in a seated position. It is a technique for releasing all the vertebrae from the top of the spine down to the 9th dorsal vertebrae. It is an excellent manipulation for freeing vertebral fixation. It uses diagonal contacts to activate the deep currents down the spine.

The head is supported by the heel of the therapist's hand under the jaw line with the fingers separated around the ear. This ensures that the head is kept in an upright position and braced against the push impulse of the thumb of the other hand along the upper vertebrae as well as centrally positioning the atlas. The arm wrapped around the clients shoulder ensures that the body does not slump forward. In this position the back is supported against your body so that the client feels safe and, being supported all round, can relax into the treatment. The arm position also enables you to move any anterior rotation of the torso back into a neutral position. The thumb pressure over the transverse process of the vertebrae is a release for the paravertebral muscles, affects the sympathetic nerve chain and can help to reposition any misaligned vertebra.

Apart form it's use on any specific single or group of painful vertebrae, when applied to all the vertebrae from the atlas down to thoracic 9 it is effective for general upper back and neck tension, headaches and for releasing gas.

I could have included this technique in the structural chapter but countryside techniques are a little bit unusual in that you are working with the body *whilst in the field of gravity* whereas most structural work is done off-gravity.

Client is seated.

1. Stand behind the client.
2. Wrap your right arm around the front of the client's right shoulder and place your right hand on the side of their head, so that the ear lies between the water and fire fingers (Fig. 49) and the ball of your left thumb at the side of a fixed and tender vertebrae.

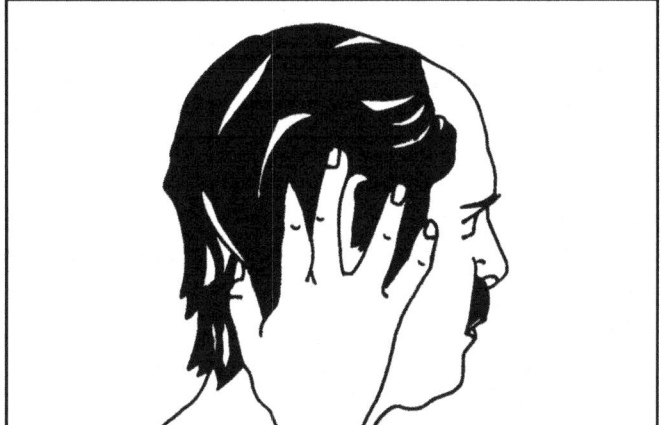

Fig. 49

3. Stimulate the vertebrae by vibrating your left thumb in towards the centre line of the body for about 1 minute, or until the tenderness has gone (Fig. 50).

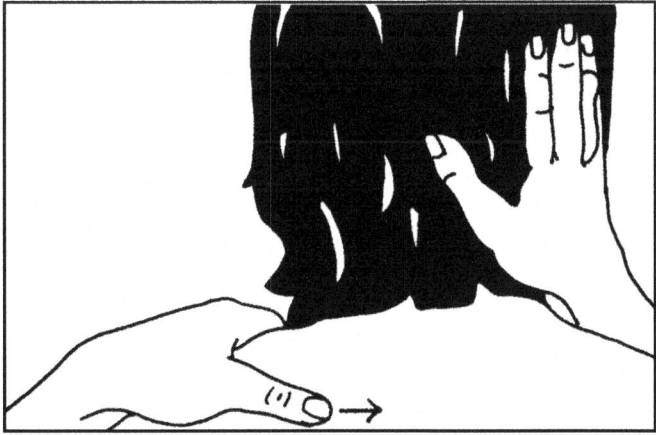

Fig. 50

4. Treat all other sore vertebrae in the same way. Treat both sides of the spine if necessary.

Lower Pelvic Release

Tension and soreness in the lower abdomen is usually indicative of disturbance in the underlying organs (the bladder, uterus, prostate, or rectum). Releasing the muscle tension above improves the functioning of the organs below. This is a strong technique and an awkward one to carry out on heavy clients but it is never the less effective in releasing muscle tension in the lower abdomen, especially the attachments of the lower rectus abdominus and pyramidalis muscles. Tension here is usually indicative of problems with the underlying organs and many bladder and uterine problems such as painful cramps during menstruation can be helped by this technique. It is not recommended during a woman's period but preferably just after menstruation has ceased.

This technique can also be used as a powerful sacral re–positioning manipulation in cases of a sacral distortion that is not reacting favourably to more gentle vibratory techniques. This variation of the technique is difficult to do and requires that general abdominal tension is fully released first with both 5-pointed star and perineal work.

Client is on their back

1. Stand on the client's right side.
2. Place your left hand underneath the back of the neck and occiput, and the ball of your right thumb flat over the tense muscle fibres just above the symphysis pubis (Fig. 51).

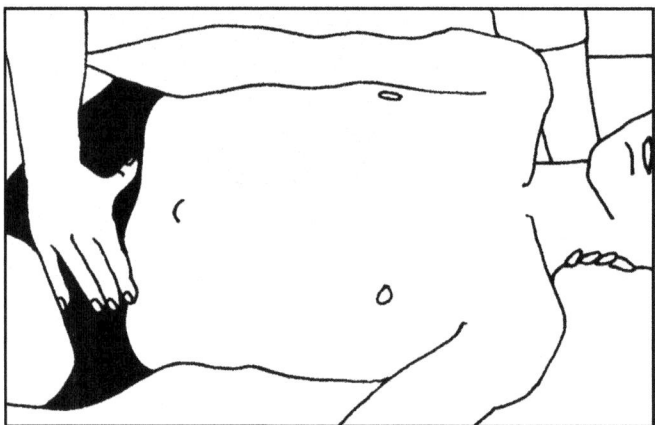

Fig. 51

3. Ask the client to breathe in, and as they breathe out lift upwards on the neck as you hold the thumb steady over the tense muscles. Hold the stretch for a moment and then let the upper body down gently. Allow a short period of relaxation and repeat the sequence three more times (Fig. 52)

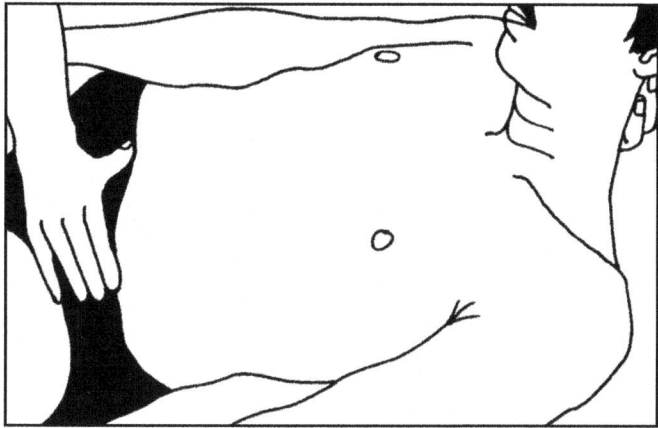

Fig. 52

N.B. When using this as a sacral correction, the thumb contact is on the anterior sacral base side of the pelvis over the middle area of the Poupart's ligament.

Stimulating Sensory Current Flow

This is an ether treatment because it works on the joints of the body. It seeks to stimulate the return or sensory flow of energy in the body from the circumference or periphery back to the centre or core, and so has a balancing effect in relation to the motor currents of energy. When Dr. Stone talks about the centre and circumference he is often referring to the umbilicus and the spirals of energy that radiates from it.

I view it as being a treatment that slows down or balances an excess of activity in the umbilical spirals of energy. The first contact points on the hands and feet are reflex points to the umbilicus. The right thumb is always 'pushing' the energy back towards the centre of the body. The left hand utilises the fire finger, so that as well as receiving energy from the right thumb, the fire finger, which has a positive charge, has a warming and opening effect *locally* on the contact points encouraging the free flow of energy through the area.

The contact areas shown in Fig. 53 are points above and below the line of flexion of a joint. Dr. Stone referred to these as 'diamond shaped areas of action.'

As the life energy crosses over through the joints making diagonal contacts across the diamond shaped areas tends to work best as these activate the deeper energy currents, though same side contacts are also used.

The session very useful in a situation where a client is pushing out far too much energy in frenetic activity; for example, in the frantic days just before Christmas. It can be done on the front or the back of the body as required.

From a symptomatic point of view, I have found this treatment to be of enormous benefit in cases of rheumatoid arthritis and for stopping the hot flushes associated with the female menopause.

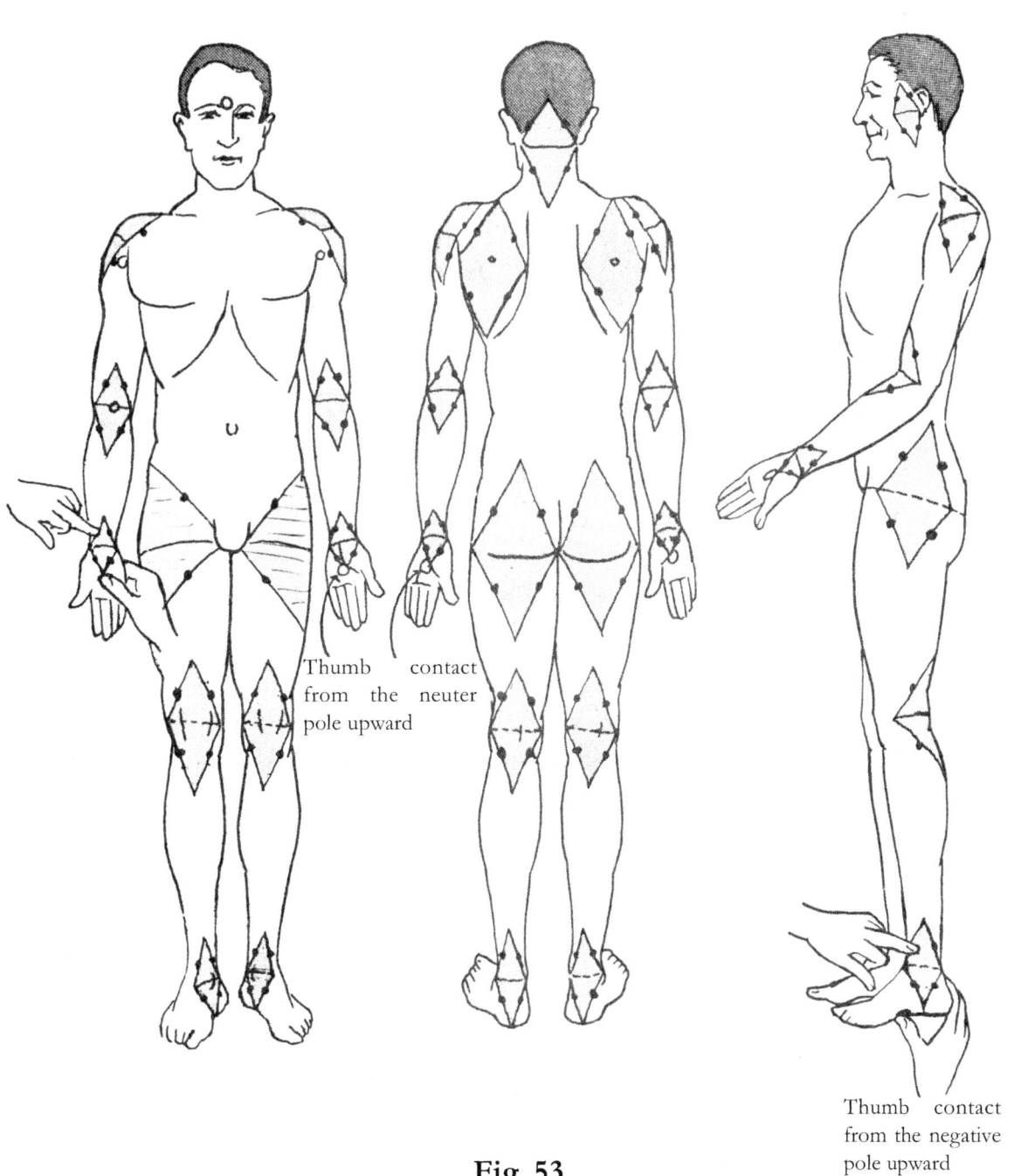

Thumb contact
from the neuter
pole upward

Thumb contact
from the negative
pole upward

Fig. 53

117

Client is on their back

1. Stand at the client's feet.
2. Place your right thumb on the sole of the right foot, and your left fire finger on one of the two lower points in the diamond–shaped pattern covering the right ankle (Fig. 54).

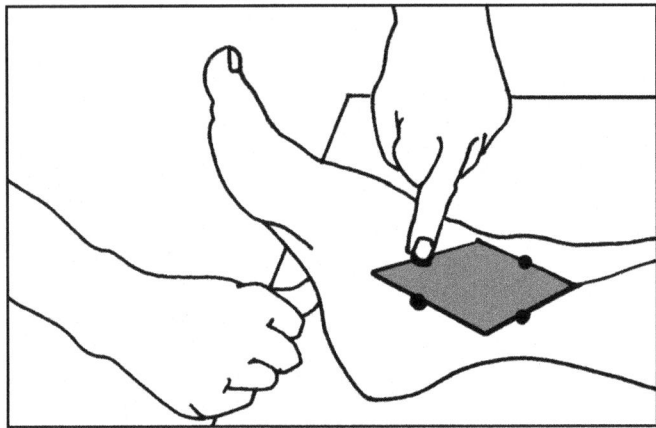

Fig. 54

3. Hold each contact area for about 1 minute until you can feel the energy strongly in the fire finger. Use gentle stimulation with the fire finger if needed.
4. Move the fire finger to one of the two upper points in the diamond over the right ankle. Move the thumb to the lower point that the fire finger has just left. (Fig. 55)

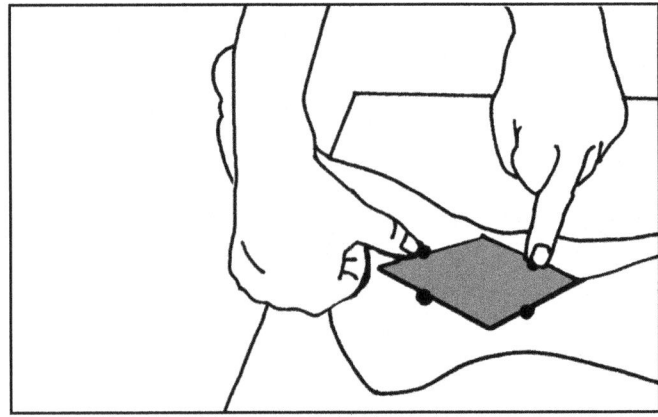

Fig. 55

5. Move the fire finger to one of the points beneath the right knee in the next diamond shape, and move the thumb to the position that the fire finger has just left (Fig. 56).

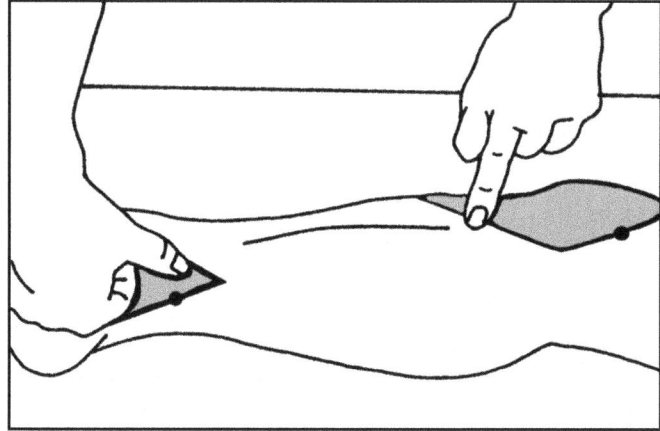

Fig. 56

6. Repeat step 3.
7. Move the fire finger to a point above the knee and the thumb to the point below it.
8. Repeat step 3.
9. Continue in this fashion until you have moved the energy above the hip joint of the right leg.
10. After coming over the right hip joint with your thumb on one of the upper points of the diamond over the hip take your left *air* finger and place it in the navel. Hold and feel for energy. This contact from upper part of hip diamond to navel finally pushes the energy from the circumference back to the centre.
11. Repeat steps 1 to 10 on the left leg and each arm. When working the arms the first contact point with the thumb is in the centre of the palm.
12. Finally, you can also push the energy back down through the jaw joint beginning with a thumb contact on the umbilical reflex on the top of the skull, near the crown. Finishing with the air finger in the navel.

Origins and Insertions Technique

This is a technique for releasing energy blocks in muscles that are manifesting as a disturbance of motor function or movement. The origin of a muscle is its point of attachment to the skeletal structure, and the insertion is the point of attachment to the bone which the muscle actually moves. The origin of the muscle is its positive pole and the insertion is the negative pole. The central body of the muscle is the neutral pole. The technique usually polarises the positive and negative poles (the origin with the insertion) however sometimes a better response comes from polarising either the positive and neutral poles or negative and neutral poles (polarising either origin or insertion with the central body of the muscle). Allow yourself to be guided by the energetic response and the relaxation of the muscle.

Releasing the Leg Muscles

This is a variation of the origins and insertion technique that specifically works the muscles in the leg. It is a general release for all the different muscles in the upper and lower leg. Stimulating the ball of the foot to encourage the air element creates energetic movement and this action on the foot also works insertions of the muscles of the lower leg whilst the other hand works behind the knee on the origins. The higher contacts around the hip and thigh influence the muscles of the upper leg.

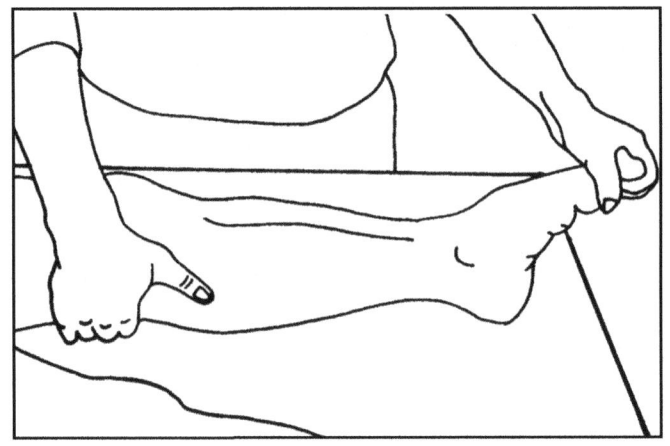

Fig. 57

1. Stand on the client's left side.
2. Place your right hand underneath the left knee from the inside of the leg. You should be able to feel numerous tendons underneath your fingers. Wrap your left hand over the left foot so that the tips of your fingers press in to the tendons around the ball of the foot (Fig. 57).
3. Stimulate alternately by pressing your fingers in to the ball of the foot, extending the toes rhythmically as you do so and using a circular movement under the back of the knee, for 2–3 minutes. Hold and feel for energy.
4. The left hand can also move to the achilles tendon area for a more specific release of the muscles in the calf, such as the gastrocnemius muscle.
5. Move the right hand up to the tendons around the hip joint and the lower spine of the ilium (Fig. 58). Alternately stimulate this area with a circular movement as you manipulate the ball of the foot for 2–3 minutes. Hold and feel for the energy

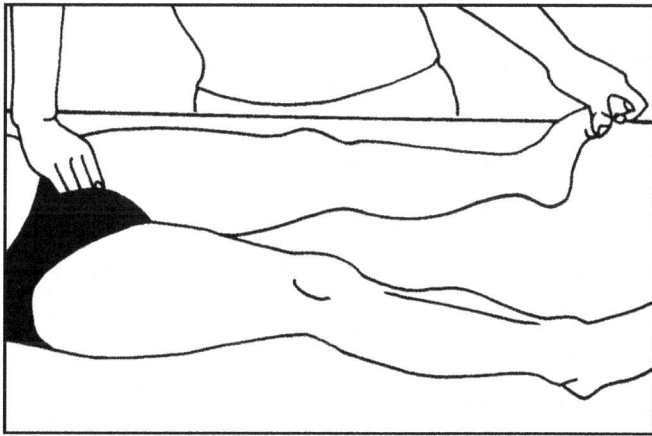

Fig. 58

Releasing the Rectus Femoris Muscle

The rectus femoris muscle is one of the quadriceps muscles in the upper leg responsible for extending the knee and straightening the leg. This muscle has been chosen simply to illustrate the basic technique. The technique can be used on any muscle, as long as you know the location of its origin and insertion.

This particlar technique can also release fire energy that has become locked in the thighs. (Fire triad: eyes/solar plexus/thighs)

Client is on their back

1. Stand on the client's left side.
2. Place the fingertips of your left hand on the tendon structure just above the patella in the middle of the leg, and the fingertips of your right hand on the origin of the muscle which is on the lower anterior iliac spine just above the position of the hip joint (Fig. 59).

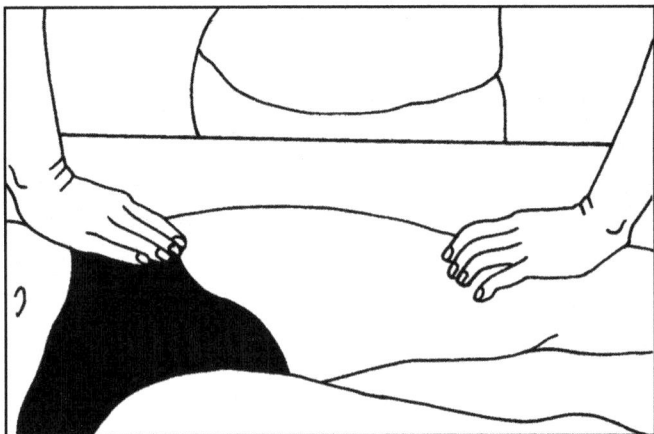

Fig. 59

3. Stimulate alternately using a circular movement of the fingertips for about two minutes. Hold and feel for energy.

Treating Pain in the Long Bones of the Legs

Pain in the long bones of the legs can indicate anaemia, lymphatic stasis, or lack of various nutrients such as vitamin C, sodium, manganese or calcium. It may also be due to exhaustion through excessive standing or walking. In many cases the roots of the pain lie in poor digestion, and should be treated with this in mind. Apart from digestive treatment local release work as set out below is also applicable.

The twisting action releases lymphatic stasis, toxic build-up and aids in re-hydrating spastic tissue. This action also has an effect on the freedom of movement of the fascia and can markedly increase the 'lift' through the structure.

Client is on their back

1. Stand on their left side.
2. Reach across their body, place your right hand on the inside of their right upper thigh and the left hand on their right lower leg (Fig. 60).

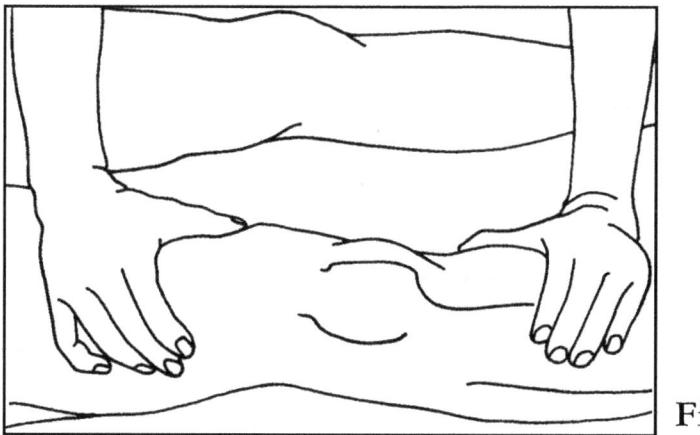

Fig. 60

3. Grip the muscles and tendons of their inner thigh and rotate your hand in an outward direction, at the same time as you grip the muscles of the lower leg and twist the tissues inwards. Vibrate your hands for about 10-20 seconds. Rest for a moment then repeat at least twice more.

4. Make other similar twisting contacts with your hands on different parts of the leg. Both contacts on the lower leg (Fig. 61) or on the upper leg.

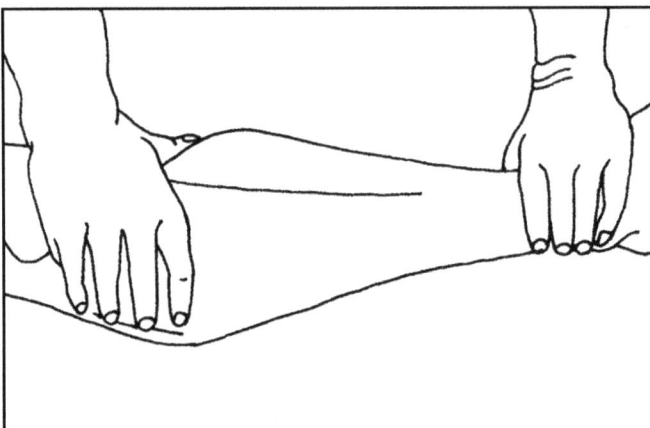

Fig. 61

5. Finally connect an outward twisting contact on the upper (or lower leg) to a contact area on the pelvis. The pelvic contact can be given either with an upward vibration or a rocking movement (Fig. 62).

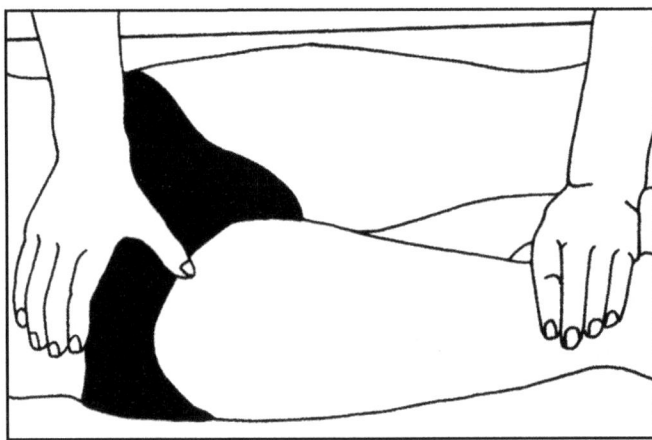

Fig. 62

8. The Art of Structural Balancing

Structural balancing refers to the aspect of the energy-balancing and bodywork that deals specifically with balancing the body's relationship to gravity. In Polarity Therapy balancing the body's relationship with gravity is considered to be the final phase of the whole energy-balancing process. It is the phase that deals with the crystallization of energy into form or matter, the physical body. Structural balancing deals with the body's relationship to external forces, in particular the force of gravity as the predominating external force acting on the body throughout its lifetime.

After more than 30 years of practising structural balancing as a major aspect of my private Polarity practice, I have moved a long way from being concerned with the mechanical perspective of level head, shoulders and pelvis, balanced sacrum and occiput and a straight spine that lies along the centre line. My primary goal is simply *comfort*. It is not crucial for health that the structure conforms to any kind of *Platonic* ideal as in a Greek sculpture of the human body. In reality, a sense of deep comfort and ease in movement are what everyone is looking for.

Oddly, there is a tendency for Polarity practitioners to polarise and separate the energetic, elemental and emotional work from the structural work as if there is no relationship between these aspects of the human being. Structural work is often viewed as working with a somewhat static process as opposed to the dynamic energy of the mind and emotions. Yet, to create true ease and comfort you need to create a relationship between both the inner and outer forces which human beings have to balance throughout life. This is not a static balance but a dynamic, fluid, ever-changing interaction. You are dealing with the client's relationship to his or her own mental and emotional centres of gravity internally as well as with the physical force of gravity externally.

Background

One of the curiosities of both teaching and practicing Polarity Therapy is that Dr. Randolph Stone, the founder of the system, began his career as an osteopath, chiropractor and naturopath; so, as a practitioner of manual medicine, structural bodywork was both his forte and his base. The students he taught Polarity Therapy to from the late 1940s through the late 1960s were all practitioners who had undergone at least three to four years of full-time training in a structural approach to manual therapy. From 1970 onwards until he retired in 1973, the students who attended his seminars had changed. They came from completely different backgrounds, being mostly reflexologists, massage therapists, Gestalt psychotherapists and body-orientated psychotherapists such as Reichians and Neo-Reichians such as Radix practitioners.

As much as Stone pursued energy—structure was his home. His first book, entitled *The New Energy Concept of the Healing Art,* and later re-issued as *Energy - The Vital Polarity in the Healing Art,* was essentially a book outlining an osteopath's journey to give the energetic model a firmer basis. Osteopathy in the era when Stone's trained (1909-1914) still had the vital life force as a one of its fundamental underlying principles. What osteopathy, at this time, did not have was a valid, clear model of where this life force came from and how it behaved. Stone laid a solid foundation for this in his first book and expanded on it over the next 15 years. In the preface to the first book, he speaks of teaching perineal and coccyx work, these being profoundly important sessions for working with structural imbalance and how, in seeking to come up with an explanation for their effectiveness, the whole of Polarity Therapy became clear to him. In this first book he also refers to "the artery rules," and "the artery rules supreme through the sympathetic nervous system." These are basic early theoretical maxims well-known to any trained osteopath:

> The rule of the artery must be absolute, universal, and unobstructed, or disease will be the result.
> *Autobiography* by A.T. Still, 1897, p. 219

> So if the supply channels of the body be obstructed, and the life-giving currents do not reach their destination full freighted, then disease sets in.
> Ibid., p.222

> The rule of artery and vein is universal in all living beings
> *Philosophy and Mechanical Principles of Osteopathy* by A.T. Still, 1892, p. 55

Simply put, the idea is that blood heals; that if you can get fresh arterial blood flowing to any part of the body it will heal. Dr. Stone also wrote "THE ARTERY RULES through this supply of Prana in the blood stream," positing a similar concept to that of Chinese traditional medicine where they say that the chi and the blood flow together.

Another basic tenet of Osteopathy is that "structure governs function." Whilst A.T. Still never said this specifically, it first appeared in one of the standard textbooks on Osteopathy:

That structure changes function must be admitted in countless cases. This fact is fundamental in osteopathic theory, according to which most diseases are either caused or maintained by structural conditions interfering with function. On the other hand, it is equally certain that in numerous cases there is evidence of the modifying influence of function on structure.

The cell doctrine as commonly understood is insufficient to explain the phenomena of the complex, organized living being. The cell represents the expression of life which in inherent in the common structural basis, protoplasm. It remains further to state, as Dr. Still himself has emphasized, that protoplasm is the **first product** of the life essence. There is an organizing force that lies back of all structure. That force is unknown but it represents an action, an energy, a function. In this sense we are justified in insisting that function is a cause of structure. We may follow out this assertion, however, with the equally obvious statement that before that organizing force can express itself in any substantial way it must have a structural basis. That structural basis is protoplasm. In this view of the matter we are justified in claiming that *structure governs function*. [Italics added.]

A Textbook of the Principles of Osteopathy by G. D. Hulett, B. S., D.O., 1903, p.25

The above quote is from the 1903 version of the book which was reprinted many times in the following decades, with various alterations to the specific text above but always ending with the same last sentence.

VITAL OR MECHANICAL

OSTEOPATHS are exercised over the question whether it is the vital mechanism or the mechanical structure that is at fault; whether the material body is capable of holding within reasonable bounds the fractious and incorrigible vital force; whether form determines function, or function determines form and in a specific case, whether the bone disturbs the muscle or whether the muscle disturbs the bone.

The Journal of Osteopathy, by G. D. Hulett, B. S., D. O., June 1901

From 1900 to 1953 osteopathic theories were modified and refined by the faculty members of several different osteopathic schools in various consensus documents. In 1922 the following tenets were stated:

1. Normal structure is essential to normal function.

2. Normal function is essential if normal structure is to be maintained.

3. Normal environment is essential to normal function and structure, though some degree of adaptation is possible for a time, even under abnormal conditions.

In 1953, Osteopathy's four fundamental principles were restated as:

1. The body is a unit.

2. The body possesses self-regulatory mechanisms.

3. Structure and function are reciprocally inter-related.

4. Rational therapy is based upon an understanding of body unity, self-regulatory mechanisms and the inter-relationship of structure and function.

Personally, I was never completely comfortable with this early simple ubiquitous statement that *structure governs function* when it was clear from my work with clients that structure and function fundamentally influence each other. Yet, my researches clearly indicated that there was a depth in the original work of A.T. Still, and his contemporaries indicated a different and deeper understanding of the interaction of structure and function. Indeed, in the writings of contemporary philosophers of science and biology, like Herbert Spencer (1820–1903) and Alfred Russel Wallace (1823–1913), the concept of the interdependence or reciprocal interrelatedness of structure and function figured strongly. I will return to the relation of structure and function later in this chapter.

It is important to remember that Dr. Stone's books were postgraduate manuals with specific relevance to doctors of manual medicine such as osteopaths and chiropractors because these were his students during the period when the five books, the set of 25 charts and assorted course notes that are now collected into Volume 1 and Volume 2 of *Polarity Therapy—the Complete Collected Works*, were written. Any recent student of Polarity

Therapy needs to bear this in mind when they are studying these volumes, as the books assume a level of underpinning knowledge that, in general, is not held by current students and practitioners of the art (2017). This is not just true of current practitioners and students but of most people who have trained in Polarity Therapy since the early 1980s when the first full practitioner trainings were created.

For example, in Volume I, Book 3, p. 66, Dr. Stone states:

> Bony adjustment and muscular stretch are structural corrections and do not always balance the energy in the POLARITY FIELDS.

Some Polarity teachers have interpreted this phrase to mean that there is no need to do structural balancing or structural correction because doing so does not always move and balance the energy. However, this is to take the comment out of context. In the quote, Stone was referring to the basic techniques of bony adjustment and muscular release technique for structural correction that was used every day by his students in their chiropractic and osteopathic work, impressing upon them the fact that such *physical* corrections do not necessarily influence the energy. He was reminding them that, no matter how evolved their manual skills were, physical manipulation did not always move the energy. In essence, what Dr. Stone was teaching was not simple physical osteopathic structural correction but energy-based correction which was a fundamentally different concept. So, to take this phrase out of context and not recognise the audience that Dr. Stone was writing for, is a grave error and has led to many trainings either completely ignoring or diluting the structural aspect of Polarity Therapy.

Early Osteopaths, Naturopaths and Chiropractors did believe that they influenced the life force or "the innate" indirectly through their manipulations. They felt that by freeing the bony articulations and relieving pressure on spinal nerves that the life force could flow again and affect the body positively. Many people in the Polarity community have, for the last 40 years, talked about Dr. Stone discovering the life force and explaining its role in manipulative therapy. It is my contention, however, that this ignores the history of manual medicine, and indeed medicine as a whole, in the eighteenth and nineteenth centuries in the USA. Chinese medicine was widely practiced from the 1870s onward throughout the Western United States. Mesmerism was widely used in the Eclectic medical schools. Joseph Rhodes Buchanan, a major figure in the history of the Eclectic medical schools, created "Sarcognomy," believing that every organ of the body is directed by a separate region of the brain by means of "nervaura," or invisible electrical currents. Dr. Stone was strongly influenced by Buchanan's work, even to the point of including some Sarcognomy charts in his own books on Polarity Therapy. The three quotes below from Buchanan are illuminating:

> ….the still more important principle that each vital function of the body and the soul is expressed at the surface of the brain and of the body, and that for every function there is an external locality at which it may be reached, and stimulated or tranquillized by nervauric methods, by electricity, or by heat, cold, and medical applications.
>
> *Therapeutic Sarcognomy* – J. R. Buchanan, 1891, Chapter 1, p. 10

> …the passage of human nervauric influence from the hand of the operator to the subject, by which so many vital influences are produced,
>
> Ibid., Chapter 3, p. 61

> …healing the human constitution by the hand, the electric poles, and the various external applications which produce different effects as they are applied to different parts of the body, for every physiological as well as every psychic function has a special portion of the surface through which it may be reached and excited.
>
> Ibid., Chapter 4, p. 72

It is my belief that what Dr. Stone really did was integrate earlier concepts that suggested that the vital life force could be influenced directly through conscious intentional touch, as it was in Mesmeric healing and Sarcognomy, and he combined it with a clear model of the manifestation and behaviour of that energy in and around the body. He did this at a time when the field of manual medicine was rushing headlong into scientific physicalism and reductionism, abandoning the concept of the vital life force and becoming more medicalised, in the sense of following the biomedical model, largely through the influence of the emerging diagnostic technologies such as x-rays and the understanding of cellular biology. In a sense, Dr. Stone did not throw out the baby with the bath water, maintaining instead a wholistic and vitalistic viewpoint, yet still being open to scientific advances particularly in the field of atomic physics.

What is Structure?

Simply put, our structure is our physical body. The shape or conformation of our structure is determined by the bony framework of the body to which is attached our musculature, connective tissue or fascia, soft tissue, organs and skin.

> In the structural field of anatomy, it is the connective tissue which is the tension factor for postural relationship and balance response, or the structural lesions in articulations and joints. Posture depends on this relationship of electromagnetic tension fields in the body structure and functional response through the life-breath, the prana currents.
>
> Vol. II, Book 6, p. 20

Dr. Stone did not often use the word "posture," tending instead to focus on the word "structure." To some extent I see structure as static and posture as dynamic. Many systems of somatic therapy focus on something that is usually referred to as good posture. Posture is the functioning of the structure. I understand good posture as the efficiency and ease with which our structure can move through its available range. Good posture is not a static thing. Posture is an often overlooked consideration in Polarity as our focus is more on the structure. The word posture also has significance in relation to our identity. Posturing or striking a pose is often related to an emotional or egoic statement.

Classically, in terms of Western anatomy and physiology, the function of the bone structure of the body is usually listed as locomotion, protection and support. Other important issues are the elasticity and flexibility of the structure. It is vital that the structure has the ability to withstand and accommodate all the compressive forces that act upon it, whether these forces are coming from the top down like gravity, or acting from the bottom up as in walking or running. It also needs a good range of movement. All of this is vital for our ability to adapt to and compensate for external forces.

There is, and has always been, a very real survival advantage of good posture. When all the parts of the body are well aligned to the vertical axis the structure of the body can be viewed as an upright cylinder. The upright human posture on two feet has a small moment of inertia in contrast to other mammals that move about on all fours. Being upright and standing on two feet gives us a capacity to make turning movements unequalled amongst mammals. The small moment of inertia inherent in good structure means that we need

131

to use very little effort to maintain our upright position and that we can turn quickly. It is probably these capabilities, inherent in a well-balanced posture, that allowed primitive man with very simple knives to either capture and kill or simply defend himself from animals much more powerful than he was.

The most efficient usage of the body's muscular energy is synonymous with having a good structure and balanced function of the structure or good posture. Good posture also permits the easy transmission of force through the structure and the inherent flexibility of a well-balanced structure gives the capacity to distort (adapt and compensate) and then bounce back.

There are many motion tests that can be integrated with the normal structural body reading that give a great deal of information as to how well the structure and its alignment supports and transmits force. However, most of these are very difficult to describe adequately in writing so we will not be exploring them here. However, a simple test that you can do that tells you something about the organisation of the body and its ability to withstand compressive force is to have a partner stand in front of you and you simply place both hands palm down on their shoulders and press downwards. The better balanced and integrated the structure the more solid the body will feel. If you try this with a number of different people, particularly those who perhaps have a pronounced sway back (extreme lumbar lordosis) you will sense a kind of weakness in the body's ability to withstand the downward pressure you exert through your hands. Do not push too hard— just strongly enough to feel the resiliency and strength of the structure as it responds to your downward pressure. If you find a partner whose structure feels very weak and spongy, take your hands away and ask them to imagine that they are just about to jump forwards with both feet together (a hop), then place your hands back on their shoulders and press down. I am almost certain that their structure will feel much stronger and more stable under your hands. If you watch the adjustments they make when shifting from their normal posture to the position where they are about to hop forward, you will learn a great deal about what adjustments might be needed to improve their structure and posture.

Crystallisation and the Structural Form of the Body

The crystallisation process that forms the physical structure occurs in much the same way a saline solution will form salt crystals if left over a period of time. In the human being this crystallisation into form is governed by the energy body, which functions as the organizing matrix. The solution from which the body is formed is the five primordial elements. The fundamental or basic structure is formed in the womb. The environment within the womb is an external factor that can profoundly influence the basic structure. Even if no structural distortion occurs pre-birth, it will almost certainly begin under the influence of all the various external factors that act from the moment of birth. Physical growth continues up to about twenty-five years of age and it is during this period that the structure changes most in a natural way due to the usual patterns of human development. During this period and continuing on through later life, all the stresses and strains both internal and external that we experience tend to cause the structure to de-form, to lose its original form. From birth, gravity and air pressure are the first physical forces that act upon the organism. Gravity is the most intense of these two primary acting forces as it is uni-directional as opposed to air pressure which is uniform all over. Gravity continues to act throughout life as a de-forming stress.

Whilst the metaphor of "crystallisation" is useful in describing the process of creation, it is less useful when it comes to trying to elucidate the dynamic process that is "life." Using the word "crystallisation" gives an all too solid and fixed image of the structure of the human body, it is actually an amazingly plastic, malleable system. You have only to compare a photograph of yourself taken today with one taken ten or twenty years ago to realize the truth of that statement. A more helpful concept when dealing with the structure and its ability to adapt are the concepts from physics known as *elastic* and *plastic deformation*.

When a sufficient load is applied to a metal or other structural material, it will cause the material to change shape. This change in shape is called deformation. A temporary shape change that is self-reversing after the force is removed, so that the object returns to its original shape, is called *elastic deformation*.

In other words, elastic deformation is a change in the shape and structure of a material when under stress that is recoverable after the stress is removed. In elastic deformation no part of the structure of the material has undergone permanent change. When the stress is sufficient to permanently deform the material, it is called *plastic* deformation. Plastic deformation of a material is permanent. One or more parts of the object under stress has undergone permanent change.

For plastic deformation to take place in a structure there will have already been the presence of elastic deformation. The release of any stressing force is concomitant with a release of elastic energy within any particular structure or system. Over time and with repeated stress the structure will release the elastic energy and change shape, but it will not return to its initial pre-stressed structure due to the plastic deformations that have occurred within it.

In terms of Polarity treatment, we often do not think about physical kinetic and elastic energies being focused on the pranic energy and its release. However, it is important to release both physical and metaphysical energies when doing structural bodywork. One of the main reasons for leaving structural work until the end of any Polarity training programme is to make sure that the student's awareness and perception of the metaphysical pranic energies is absolutely clear and stable so that when beginning to use the more physical stretch-release techniques of structural work, engaging the kinetic and elastic energies, that the awareness of the prana is not lost. It is all too easy when doing structural bodywork, which involves the intelligent use of a certain amount of physical strength, to lose contact with the life energy and end up doing a simple manual, rather than Polarity, treatment.

Structure as Identity

For me, the true significance of structural work is that, at a fundamental level, structure is identity. We can recognise a friend some hundreds of metres away in a crowd, just by the set of their neck and shoulders and the way they move, even though their back may be to us. There is a unique individuality and expression of personal identity in the way we hold our body and in the way in which we move.

One of the reasons we have such individuality of structure is the length of time it takes a human being to learn to stand and walk. Typically, it takes some 12-18 months for a baby to achieve these abilities. Some will develop quicker than others but it is one of the longer apprenticeships in the mammalian kingdom in terms of the development of the skill of movement. A foal or calf will be able to stand and walk within one to two hours from birth. A puppy will take some five to six weeks before it can walk. The longer the time period it takes for a mammal to move, the more individuality it will have in terms of its posture and gait. If you own a black cat and put it in a field with 50 other black cats of similar size about 100 metres away, you will be very hard pressed to pick out which cat is yours because they will all move and stand in much the same way. Yet we would have no problem picking out a friend or partner in a crowd much further away, as there is a huge diversity in human posture and movement, a uniqueness that is easily visible.

Most people believe that we show our ego, our identity, through our words and emotional expression; yet, when looking in the mirror, we often speak of *seeing our self*. It is not our egoic self in terms of mind, emotions and character that we see in the mirror, but its expression through our structure. In some sense, our primary experience of our self, our identity, only happens when we see ourselves in a mirror or perhaps on a video. That experience is immediate and is based upon our visual perception of our structure and what it says about us long before any words may emerge.

In some cultures, the ego was considered to be a shadow structure, in as much as it was only visible when forced to react to some situation; the light of interaction delineating the ego as a shadow on the screen of life. As soon as the interaction is over the ego disappears. I am reminded of the spiritual teacher Osho saying that it was very easy to love yourself when you live in a cave on a mountain as there is little to expose your ego but that the real challenge was to maintain that good feeling about yourself whilst in a relationship where your ego is being constantly provoked and revealed. Yet, if structure is identity, there is never actually a time when it is invisible either to you or to others. Your structure and your identity, as it expresses itself through it, is a constant presence. You don't even have to look at yourself in a mirror. You can catch a glimpse of yourself reflected in another's eye.

Structure as Relationship

Structure is also about relationship. One of the primary forces that we are in relationship to throughout our whole life is the force of gravity but we also have a relationship with the world at large as well as our more personal human relationships.

Gravity begins to influence us as soon as we leave the womb and the buoyancy of the amniotic fluid that surrounds us in utero. At this point we are also in immediate and direct relationship with our mother and father. These primary relationships and others continue throughout life and, to greater or lesser extent, we adapt our structure to compensate for the impact these forces exert upon us. For most people identity is synonymous with an egoic sense of self which is something that is developed over years from the moment we are born. Up until the point at which a child's sense of self and ego becomes somewhat crystallised the structure is more balanced. In the young child, the spine is straighter as there is minimal impact from internal forces as the nascent ego is more fluid and undeveloped. Their inherent alignment is almost perfect. Then, as they learn to stand and walk, beginning their exploration of movement in the field of gravity, their ability to elastically adapt to gravity as the major external physical force that will affect them throughout their life is at such a maximal level that the structure is hardly compromised.

Of course, in some families a young child can experience major challenges in its relationship with its parents. Some children in this situation will introject the difficulties in this primary relationship into their ego structure and that will create a cascade of changes and adaptations that will significantly alter their structural balance. It is quite possible that another sibling in the same family may have far less imbalance in their structure as they may have found a way to discharge the impact of the parental dynamic. As soon as a young child enters the school system, he or she begins to experience other powerful relationships with both peers and teachers. It is at this stage that more and more structural imbalance becomes evident as his or her identity changes and grows, shaped by these relationships.

Gravity

Human beings have evolved over millions of years within the field of gravity. We are intrinsically designed to cope with gravity as an external force. Our awareness of any constant force, such as air pressure or gravity, that exists around us or influences us is screened out like any constant input into our body. Just the same way in which, after a while, a person living near an airport or train station does not hear the planes or trains. Generally, there has to be a rise in the threshold of the incoming signal for us to be aware of it. Air pressure, just like gravity, is a constant on the body from the moment of birth and it exerts a quite considerable force on the body (14.7 pounds per square inch or 101 kPa) yet, because it is spread over the whole body, we have no need to adapt to it as it exerts equal force on us in all directions; nor are we even aware of it except in circumstances such as a sudden drop in air pressure due to an approaching storm front or perhaps at very high elevations where the pressure is much less than at sea level.

We all know what gravity is and this is very simply expressed in the phrase "that which goes up must come down." Most people will remember from studying science at school that gravity is the force that pulls things towards the centre of the Earth and that it acts at right angles to the surface of the Earth. The word gravity is used quite a lot in everyday life. It has both literal and metaphorical meanings. Gravity is an invisible force that we only know through its effect. Most people know that somehow gravity is related to the experience of weight and that when gravity is not active as, for example, when an astronaut is so far away from the earth that gravity is no longer an influence, the astronaut experiences weightlessness. Our weight is actually the mass of our body times the force of gravity.

So, although gravity is a constant force, we do have an awareness of it through its action in the creation of our weight. Our experience of our weight is variable because some things can alter the effect of gravity on the mass of our body. Our most common experience of weight change is when we are in water, either in the sea, a swimming pool or in a bath where the buoyancy of the water partially counteracts the force of gravity. I often recommend to students that the next time they take a bath they continue to lie in it as the water drains away and experience the gradually increasing effect of gravity as the water level drops. It is an interesting experience to feel the increase in weight and to get a sense of just how strong gravity and its effect upon structure is.

Even without the effect of water most people will have had the experience of their weight changing. Some days you can get up in the morning feeling light and almost weightless, experiencing your movements being free and easy. On other days, you can get up and feel tired and extremely heavy, hardly being able to lift your body up from the bed, experiencing what some people have called "heavy gravity," meaning that it is as if the force of gravity has increased somehow. In this scenario, your movements feel lethargic and you hardly have the energy to put one foot in front of the other. On these days it feels as if gravity is exerting a stronger pull on your body. Actually, it's not gravity that is changing, as it is constant, but your relationship to it has changed profoundly because of an alteration in your own internal gravity.

> The earth's gravity force does not rule man. It only conditions him when his own gravity fields are out of balance. Man is an integral unit, having a central gravity line of force of his own by which he acts and around which his forces spin as the central orbit of his being.
>
> Vol. I, Book 3, p. 64

The idea that you have your own *internal centre of gravity,* as Stone indicates above, requires some deeper exploration. The idea of a centre of gravity unrelated to the physical pull of the earth is perhaps most widely used in the military. In this context it is often used in reference to strategic planning around the enemy's centre of gravity. In a general physical sense, the centre of gravity of an object is the point at which a force applied to it will move it most efficiently. Pushing through the centre of gravity involves the most economical usage of energy when applied and done with sufficient force to cause an object to lose balance and topple over. We could say that centre of gravity in any structure or system is that part or aspect that has the required centripetal force to hold the structure together. So, in military terms, attacking the enemy at their centre of gravity is the place that is most likely to result in their defeat.

A person's internal centre of gravity is the axis around which their whole life revolves. It is that which holds the person together mentally and emotionally and gives resilience. The beliefs, attitudes and deeply held values around which a person's life revolves are the person's internal centre of gravity. A person's whole life could revolve around one single, deeply-held attitude or belief about oneself, such as the concept of loyalty. This kind of belief exerts a centripetal force that literally holds the person together psychologically. It is quite possible to have more than one internal centre of gravity and for it to shift and change over time. An organising value that worked when the person was in his or her twenties and early thirties may not exert the same kind of pull when the person reaches forty. As higher frequency energies, these kinds of attitudes, beliefs and values have a powerful organising effect on the movement of the prana in the energy body. Any life experience or internal doubt or intellectual challenge could significantly alter a person's centre of gravity, destabilising it dramatically. If this happens, the ramifications ripple through the energy body into the structure of the physical body. Some people have constantly changing centres of gravity, some of which enhance the integrity of the physical structure and others which destabilise it. In the human body there is a connection between where the centre of gravity is physically and the centre of balance. The same is true of our internal gravity and internal psychological balance. Balance in the human being is more about dynamic instability or unstable equilibrium than it is about static balance. You could say we dance in an ever-changing relationship between internal and external gravity.

Any energy balancing work with a client can affect the person's internal centres of gravity. This will always have some impact upon the person's relationship to external physical gravity and is why I have often said that all Polarity treatments are structural. This is a concept I will return to later in this chapter when we explore body reading and structural treatment.

As gravity is a force or pull acting at right angles to the Earth's surface, its effect is greatest on us when we are standing. In standing, gravity pulls down through the whole of our body. Initially, when lying down, being largely "off gravity," our physical body and its muscular holding relates to our inner mental and emotional balance, our internal centres of gravity, establishing what I call *intrinsic structural alignment*. Once we stand upright, we have a primary adaptation of this intrinsic alignment to the force of gravity, followed more or less immediately by secondary compensations caused by other internal and external stresses, be they emotional, mental, energetic or physical. We can then experience tertiary and quaternary compensations caused by further stresses. Our fundamental adaptation to gravity is a measure of how well our physical structure reacts to another force, be it physical or mental-emotional, in addition to all our pre-existing internal stresses and strains.

Gravity is the major external force acting on the body. It is not the only one; but as it is the major one, the way in which the body deals with it is a metaphor for the way in which all other external forces are dealt with. Most of the general, elemental and neurological energy-balancing in Polarity Therapy deals with inner relationships, e.g. the relationship between the mind, emotions and the vital physiological functioning and how they affect our internal gravity.

> The person's own center of gravity in relation to his inner forces is <u>far more important</u> than the center of gravity outside.
>
> Vol. I, Book 3, p. 63

Structural balancing deals with outer relationships, e.g. the body's relationship with gravity, but also in a much broader sense with the life as a whole; human relationships; work; leisure activities and so on. The way a client organizes themselves in relation to gravity tells a great deal about the way in which they deal with life. The degree to which a client's body distorts in relation to gravity also tells you the degree to which they distort in relation to all other external factors. The impact of intimate personal relationships can be considered as the next major force acting on us after gravity.

Energy and Structure

What is the relationship between the energy and the structure? The first point to understand is that it is the muscles that determine the bony alignment of the structure; to be specific, the balance of muscular tension or tonus between the various groups of muscles. What, then, is the relationship between the muscles and the life energy? We all know just how profoundly our posture and therefore our muscular tension changes in relation to our state of being. Think back to the last time you felt happy and joyful, I can guarantee that you stood taller, straighter and moved far more easily than normal. What about a time when you felt depressed? I have no doubt that some combination of the following things occurred: your diaphragm tensed up, your breathing became shallow and your lumbar curve decreased, giving you a rounded lower back; your shoulders slumped, your neck collapsed and so on. The link between the muscles and the life energy is clearly the emotions.

We cannot speak of emotions without understanding that mind and emotions work together. Mind both in the sense of memory and thought process has a great deal of effect on the emotions in the sense of either inhibiting or reinforcing the emotional energy. Any disturbance to the free flow and expression of emotion can result in a pattern of muscular tension that is often referred to as body "armouring," our experience of which is part of our identity. Emotional disturbances and their related patterns of muscular armouring make it impossible for the body to adapt in an efficient way to the external force of gravity. This relationship of energy to structure is part of the step-down or involutionary phase of energy movement, during which consciousness and energy manifest into physical form.

To a large extent this step-down process informed most of my early thinking about structural bodywork but over many years and after many hundreds of structural sessions, I began to focus more and more on the evolutionary or step-up phase of energetic movement. During this time, I was also deeply influenced by the writings of Gregory Bateson, particularly in the realm of cybernetics. As I pondered the whole process of energetic movement from source to body and the return to source, I began to see the whole process as one that was governed by many complex positive and negative cybernetic feedback loops operating at many levels. Positive feedback loops amplify change; this tends to move a system away from any specific state of equilibrium and hence make it less stable. Negative feedback loops dampen or inhibit change; this tends to make a system more stable.

For example, a person has a specific weight which he or she wants to maintain, i.e., a state of stable equilibrium relating to their weight. They eat a piece of chocolate cake and like the experience at an emotional level and so eat more and more. This is a positive emotional feedback loop that reinforces their behaviour. They end up being far from their desired weight. Alternatively, the same person eats some chocolate cake, likes it and goes to have another piece but remembers wanting to maintain the desired weight and decides

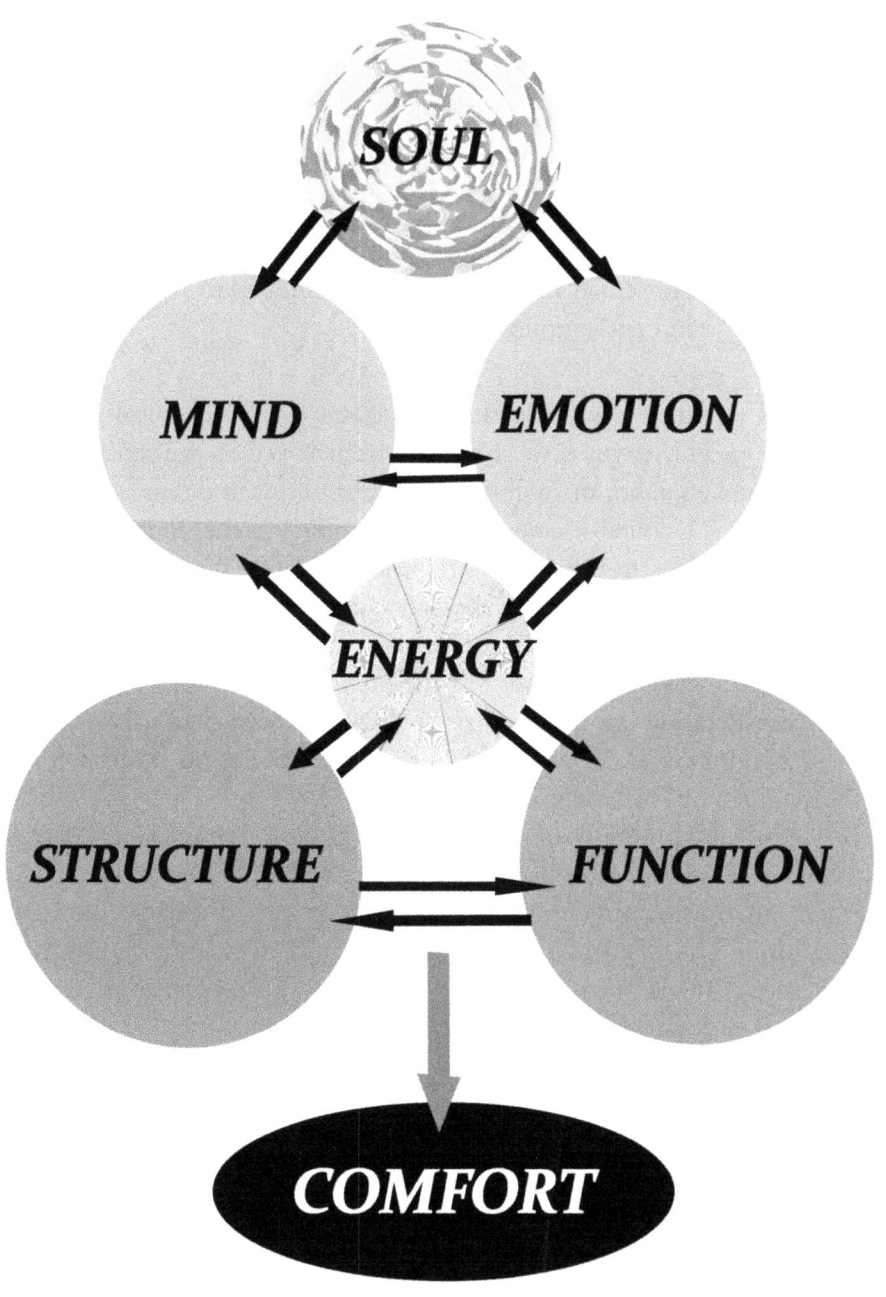

Fig. 63

against it. This is a negative mental feedback loop that limits behaviour. Thus, he or she maintains the desired weight.

The interaction between all the aspects of a human being as a set of complex feedback loops is shown in Fig.63 (on previous page). It speaks to the basic concept of the soul manifesting comfortably and easily in the world.

As I mentioned earlier, the phrase "structure governs function" is an early osteopathic maxim that was modified later to "structure and function are interrelated." In the article excerpt overleaf you can see an early osteopath wrestling with the relationships between structure, function, mind and emotion:

> But it is manifestly possible that influences not mechanical may cause fluctuations in the vital level. Impulses transmitted to the sensorium may disturb vital equilibrium. Will this condition result in disease? Fluids seek their level. The vital element is comparable to the fluid. Emotional, mental, or other non-material influence disturbs the fluid level. Vital equilibrium is lost. Removing the stimulus restores that equilibrium and the self-regulative capacity of vitality becomes apparent. In this disturbance of vital level, we find the only basis for mind therapy. From this consideration we may explain a few acute diseased conditions, and these conditions are self-limited, hence treatment is not indicated other than the removal of the exciting influence.
> But another condition may arise. Take a case in which the exciting influence is emotion. Let that emotion be continuous. Disturbed vital level reacts on organic function. Ultimately we find a disturbed mechanical condition. The disturbed physiology initiated through non-mechanical influence is made permanent (chronic) through mechanical influence. In this case mechanical treatment is indicated.
> We have said that in disturbed physiological conditions not associated with mechanical lesion mechanical treatment is not indicated. Why? Vitality is not a force to be tampered with other than by securing freedom for its action. Given unobstructed freedom self-regulation is sufficient. Granting that we possibly can hasten the process of readjustment we may not do so with ultimate benefit to the individual. Stimulation of a function beyond its normal limits under existing circumstances is a detriment. Stimulation for the sake of the exhilarating effect it produces results in the treatment

habit which in one sense is as pernicious as the drug habit. Given a correct mechanical alignment the self-regulative power of vitality becomes the all-efficient and the all-sufficient physician.

Vital or Mechanical by G. D. Hulett, B. S., D. O.
The Journal of Osteopathy, June 1901

Working with a simple command and control mechanism, as a therapeutic process, is covered by the familiar osteopathic phrase *find it, fix it, leave it alone*. In Polarity Therapy, I see the therapeutic work on body structure as our interaction with all the multiple positive and negative feedback loops between, soul, mind, emotions, energy, structure and function rather than any form of alteration or modification of a simple command and control mechanism.

As much as structure governs function, function influences structure. In Polarity theory much is made of triads or triune function so we can expand this and say that a balanced interaction of structure and function creates ease and comfort. Adding the element of energy to the equation creates another layer of triadic interaction. This can be articulated as energy influences both structure and function and that structure and function both affect the energy. Yet, energy itself is influenced by still higher levels of structure and function, these being mind and emotion. We can go even higher in the vibratory realm above mind and emotion and speak of soul influencing mind and emotion and being influenced by all the other elements in this complex interacting system.

Every human being will have some aspects of oneself more dominant and pathways within this complex feedback system more active. Some will use more negative inhibitory feedback loops, others will use positive amplifying feedback. Some will use positive feedback at one level and negative at others. Some will have their mind influence their energy, which will directly influence their function, without their structure being part of the process at all. Others will have mind influence energy, which will impact their structure directly without much impact on function. The interaction between structure and function is crucial to the emergence of a sense of comfort, but this expression at the lowest level of the chart is influenced by all the other feedback loops above it. Test all the feedback loops shown in Fig. 63 against any client that you know well and it will give you invaluable insight into specific treatment strategies to adopt and help you to understand all the things that are causing the structural imbalance they are manifesting.

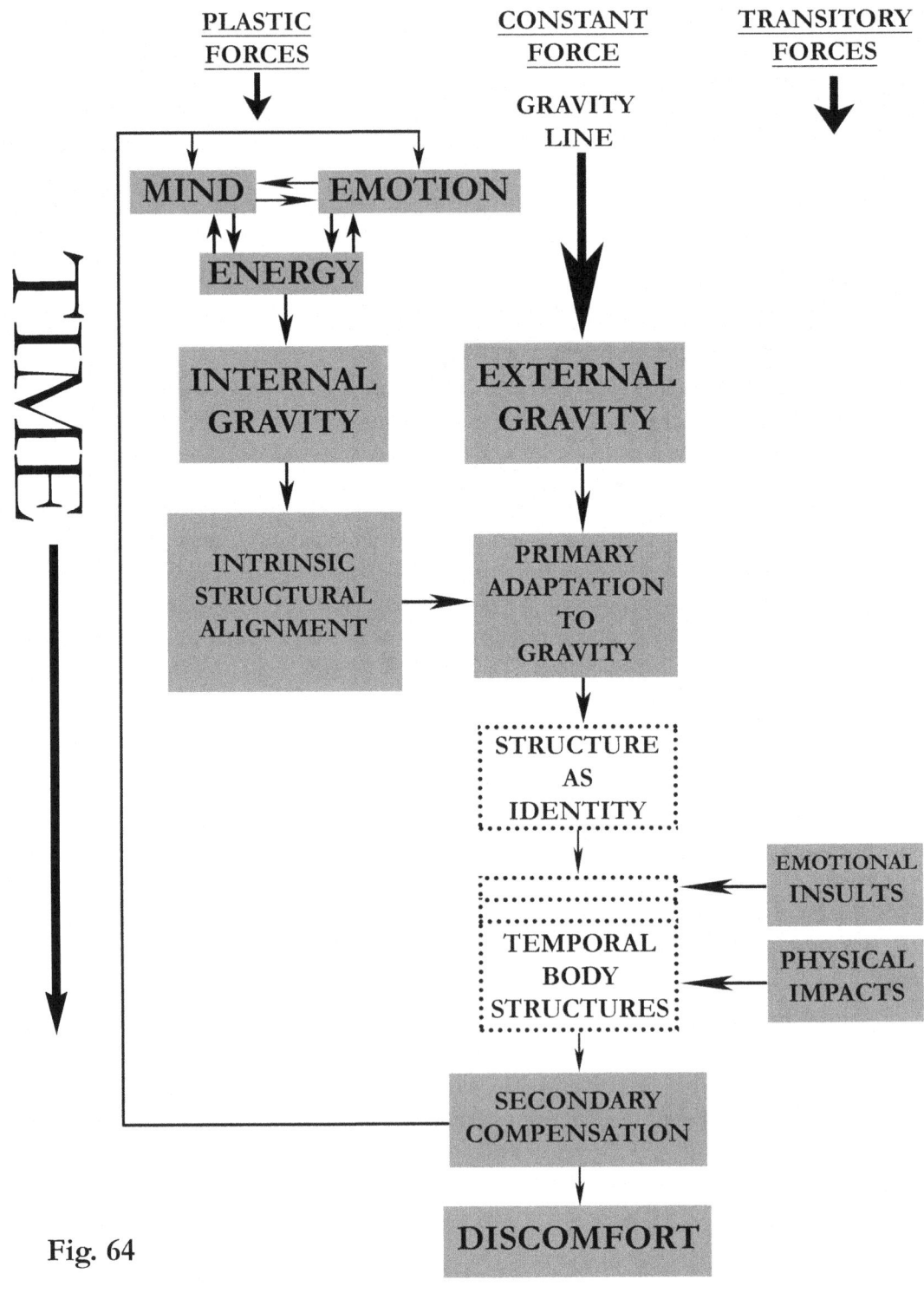

Fig. 64

144

I would suggest that the situation is actually even more complex than Fig. 63 implies. Earlier I shared a quote from Dr. Stone on p. 139 where he indicated the greater importance of a person's relationship to their inner centre of gravity over the outer physical one and expanded on the concept when I was discussing the force of gravity. The particular pattern of thoughts, beliefs, values and emotions that constellate together to form a person's internal "sun" or centre of gravity around which their whole life revolves is what primarily affects the person's intrinsic structural alignment, see Fig. 64. This is the alignment of their body before any extrinsic forces act upon it. The degree of balance within this intrinsic alignment and its inherent level adaptability and pliability is crucial to how well the structure copes when extrinsic forces come into play.

As an example, a person wakes up in the early morning and takes a moment to luxuriate in the warmth of the bed and the sunlight filtering through the windows. The person feels good to be alive. At this stage their mind and emotions are in a balanced harmonious state and their intrinsic body alignment will reflect that as they lie there in bed. The structure will be quite balanced. Physical gravity as an extrinsic force will be minimally impacting the body as it is only acting though short cross-sections of the body, as opposed to pulling through the long axis of the body (See the arrows in fig. 65).

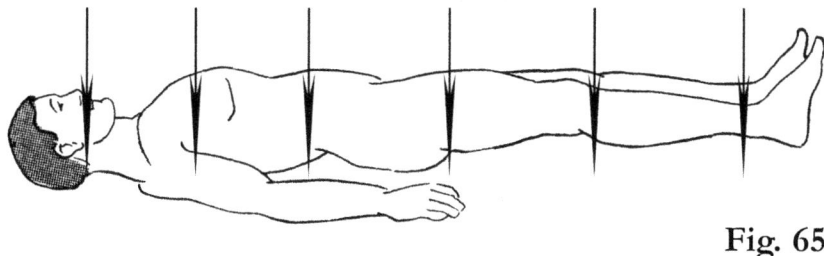

Fig. 65

When the person stands up and gravity immediately begins to affect the alignment of the body, pulling down through its long axis, what is manifest then is the person's primary structural adaptation to gravity. In this orientation, as the intrinsic alignment is balanced, their primary adaptation to gravity is also balanced and the person experiences a degree of ease and comfort as one washes, dresses and moves through the day.

However, there are days when this same person awakens and perhaps experiences an immediate sense of anxiety upon thinking about completion of a difficult project at work or payment of the monthly bills. This mental/emotional/energetic disturbance alters the internal centre of gravity, and the intrinsic alignment is no longer balanced. Even before arising, the person's body will have lost some of its innate adaptability. The possibility of a fluid, primary adaptation to gravity is compromised. In this case, the person arises and immediately feels aches in various muscles as the body reacts to gravity. The individual may even have some fleeting thoughts of feeling their age, which itself affects their internal centre of gravity even more.

Then, perhaps an hour later, just before the person in this example must leave the house to go to work, he or she decides to move a heavy piece of furniture or perhaps accidentally drops their keys behind the kitchen table. Either of these actions requires a lot of muscular activation involving lifting and/or twisting. As the person acts there is a sudden feeling of something in their back reacting. Sudden, severe pain and loss of mobility mark the start of secondary compensations as these compensatory mechanisms alter the individual's structure to try and limit the pain and discomfort. As the affected individual experiences the physical effects of this compensatory shift in body alignment, their mind fills with images all the possible ramifications of the injury in both a practical and emotional sense. This "alarm bell" of imagined ramifications is "heard" by the mind and emotions, causing further shifts of structure as their internal gravity changes, affecting the intrinsic alignment even more, causing even more compensations relative to gravity. These are called secondary, tertiary and quaternary compensatory patterns, and there can be more.

Most of these patterns will be based at a physical level on negative feedback loops that are functioning to take the structure away from pain and back into some sense of comfort. However, at a mental and emotional level, there could be many positive feedback loops that are taking the system even further away from comfort, perhaps because the person needs a rest from the challenges of work and the back pain could allow this person to take sick leave. There could even be conflict between positive emotional loops and negative mental loops, thus adding to the layers of compensation and even deeper complexity, because some of these mental and emotional loops may be operating well outside of any conscious awareness.

Structure as History

Time is an interesting factor in this model. In a sense, as much as we have a physical body as well as an energy body, we also have mental and emotional structures. Some would call these mental and emotional structures "bodies" also. Beyond them, I would suggest we have a temporal body. This is a body governed by the so-called arrow of time, the movement of time from the present moment into the future that leaves the past in its wake.

In the same sense as the ancient Greek philosopher Zeno of Elea described a paradox of time and motion by asking this intriguing question: When speaking of the flight of an arrow, if at any single *instant* the arrow can be considered to be stationary by occupying a space equal to itself, when does it move? In exactly the same way, we too can consider when does the human body actually move, change and adapt? We know that it does, but when do the changes in the structure take place? Do they take place in an instant? But then when does the next shift take place? An instant later? Part of the key to resolving Zeno's paradox lies in the definition of *an instant in time*. I do not intend to explore this further, except to say one of the benefits of considering any kind of paradox is the way it makes you think outside of any familiar framework or box. I will just ask, could we not have an unending series of temporal bodies?

When we do a structural reading of the body our consciousness is taking a snapshot in time of a temporal body. A snapshot of a body that is normally in constant motion, changing and adapting all the time. Some of these patterns of compensation become fixated in the structure as a snapshot of the compensations at a particular moment in life. A moment of frozen time expressed in and through the structure.

The patterns of compensation in the body build up over time, like layers of an onion or growth rings in a tree, as illustrated in Fig. 66. So, in two senses we can say that structure is history: first, by the way in which compensations express themselves in the body as a sort of snapshot in time; and, second, in the way in which these compensations "build up" in "layers" over time.

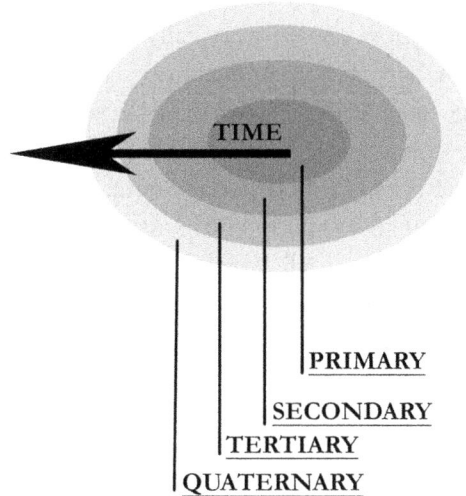

TIME

PRIMARY
SECONDARY
TERTIARY
QUATERNARY

Fig. 66

147

Postural Equilibrium

Many compensatory patterns emerge due to physical pain or injury. These patterns tend to be a combination of the body's natural tendency to immobilize a damaged area to prevent further injury, combined with trying to find a position which minimises the pain. However, a large percentage of structural imbalance in the form of compensatory patterns tends to be small, layered deviations. If you consider such everyday phrases as "being level-headed," "being on the level," "front and centre," "being off one"s rocker," "bending the truth," "the straight and narrow," "facing up to things," "dealing with things head on," "being upfront," "squaring off," "he is a square," it is obvious that there is some kind of geometry of the horizontal and vertical that underpins our identity and way of being in the world emotionally, mentally and physically. This is, at least in part, the basis of the ideal posture of the level head and pelvis and a spine that is on the centre line that I mentioned at the beginning of this chapter. The orientation of our head in space is crucial to good posture.

The equilibrium of our standing posture is fundamentally related to the maintenance of a horizontal and vertical eye line through the visual sense. The inner ear mechanism is another important mechanism in the maintenance of the standing posture. This balance mechanism also works in both horizontal and vertical planes just as vision does, but it is a less sensitive and hence less accurate system. The other key part of maintaining postural balance is our kinaesthetic sense or sensory appreciation of our body's orientation in space.

All of these three mechanisms work together to help create postural equilibrium through keeping the head in balanced position. When physically injured, it is interesting to note that blind people have fewer simple compensations than sighted people. Their compensatory patterns being just based upon the vestibular apparatus and the kinaesthetic sense. Of all the three ways in which the neurology works to maintain postural balance the kinaesthetic sense is the least accurate. It is this lack of accuracy in the body's kinaesthetic sense that causes many compensatory shifts. You can do a little experiment that is instructive. Find a small weight (about 12 ounces or 400 grams), perhaps something like a medium-size paperback book and hold it in your right hand. Now stand up and put your arms straight out in front of you, using your eyes to make sure they are both perfectly level and parallel to the ground. Now close your eyes and lift the right hand up with the weight until the arm is at a 45-degree angle to the ground. Hold it for a slow count of twenty. Keep your eyes closed. Then bring your arm down level with your other arm again, making sure that they *feel* completely level. Now open your eyes and I would be greatly surprised if they were actually level even though you felt they were! Your eyes are now telling you something quite different, the right arm being slightly higher than the left. Now make your arms level. Then put the weight down and relax. It seems you can't fully trust the accuracy of your bodily kinaesthetics but that you can trust your own eyes.

It has been well recognised within the bodywork community, particularly by teachers of the Alexander Technique, that our sensory perception is for most people quite faulty. It is even more so when the system is loaded with even quite a small amount of mechanical stress as the exercise above demonstrated. It is possible to train the kinaesthetic sense to be more accurate, and in general dancers and athletes have better sensory appreciation than the average person, but to train it to a high level of accuracy requires more dedication than most people are willing to undertake.

To get a sense of how the structure distorts after a small injury, imagine that while standing in a queue someone steps back, accidentally treading down on the instep of the right foot of the person behind. This moves out of position at least one of the cuneiform bones that help to create the arch in the foot. It is a little painful and affects the lower leg so that the ankle feels collapsed and the knee is twisted inward slightly. This will throw the right side of the pelvis and chest forward. Then, because everyone tends to squarely face the direction in which they are going to move, there is a self-correcting impulse whereby the torso is rotated back on the right so that the chest is facing front. Due to the inaccuracy of the kinaesthetic sense, what often happens is that the torso moves back on the right a little too far, and this means the head is now turned slightly to the right and so another automatic correction takes place in the neck, based upon the visual feedback, so that the eyes face front. Now there is a fully compensated pattern in the structure, a secondary set of compensations that are overlying the primary adaptation to gravity.

You can mimic this type of injury right now by standing and letting your right ankle collapse inward slightly and also allowing your knee to turn inward, you will then feel how this makes your pelvis move forward on the right. Now, while maintaining the collapse in the ankle and the inward rotation of the knee, create a compensatory movement to pull the pelvis back from its right-side-forward position to help square it up so that it faces front again, almost inevitably you will slightly overdo the movement and you will now find that your head is facing slightly to the right, so compensate for that by turning your head so that it is again squarely facing front. If you do all this, then I am certain you will feel a lot muscular tension in your body. Your knee will feel uncomfortable and you will feel tension in your mid- and lower-back muscles, and perhaps pain even in your neck.

In the case of an actual injury of this type, when the compensation is held for quite some length of time while waiting for the injury to heal, some of the other feedback mechanisms mentioned earlier will come into play and alter the structural alignment to seek some greater ease and comfort in the body. Physically, this might involve some overall weight shift to the side that is not damaged—a lateral translation of the body. This would be tertiary compensations laid over the top of the secondary ones. Then all that is needed would be another injury or further shift in your internal gravity for there to be a further ongoing series of compensatory patterns laid on top of the secondary and tertiary compensations. It really is very much like the layers of an onion, all of which have to be peeled away to get back to a more neutral primary adaptation to gravity (see Fig. 66).

The Ideal Body Pattern

In Dr. Stone's formulation of structural work, he clearly followed a bio-mechanical model of the ideal body pattern (Fig. 92, p. 189). As I mentioned at the beginning of this chapter, I initially followed this concept but then abandoned it in favour of the creation of comfort. So, what is the relevance of this image of the structure in which the spine is the centre line and the head, shoulders and pelvis are all level? In my early bodywork practice I worked to this model. While it occasionally seemed achievable, and the client experienced more ease and comfort, more often than not I came nowhere near achieving this kind of ideal pattern. I was almost always able to relieve my clients' pain and increase their comfort and sense of ease in their body so that, in their own terms, the structural issues had been entirely resolved. However, most were nowhere close to the ideal pattern. Then, in my continuing study of Dr. Stone's work, I noticed the quote below:

> Many people go around humpbacked and all distorted, and live to a ripe old age. It is not the structure that kills us, but the vital function's inability to act. True, every organ must have room in which to expand and contract; but correcting a visible, external distortion does not necessarily correct a vital function.
>
> Vol. II, Book 5, p. 59

In this comment, he clearly calls into question the therapeutic value of an ideal body pattern. If the structure is reducing the space for organs to function effectively, then structural correction is clearly vital. However, as he says, correcting the structure does not necessarily mean that you are going to be correcting impaired physiological functioning.

I quickly realised that I could do structural work that created a sense of ease and comfort and cope with the anomaly of not getting my clients to conform to the ideal model. Nevertheless, it was an internal conflict. Later, when I began teaching the structural aspect Polarity to students, I felt I had to resolve this conflict. I read extensively on other structural approaches that dealt with gravity and structure, such as Rolfing and its offshoots like Hellerwork and Postural Integration. I also explored the work of John Hurley, DC and Helen Sanders, DC, initially called Aquarian Age Healing and Applied Bio-mechanics, later renamed Spinal Touch, as well as going back to early osteopathic theories. Hurley's work was particularly interesting because his system also used the gravity board and clearly espoused the ideal viewpoint and focus on the sacrum. I also explored what you could call the epistemology and ontology that underpins the whole field of structural bodywork. I found the writings of Don Hanlon Johnson particularly helpful in this regard.

After much study and reflection, I was finally able to completely abandon the ideal model in favour of a more organic approach oriented towards the creation of comfort that is deeply respectful of a client's unique *structural expression*. The simple way I explain this to students is to call their attention to the natural world, usually referring to a forest of trees, pointing out that we do not walk into a forest and, in looking at the huge variety of shape and structure that trees express individually, say that any particular tree is flawed or in need of re-shaping. We just accept that unique expression of *treeness*. We do realise that some trees may be more vulnerable to physical forces such as wind, because of the way they have grown, but that does not necessarily impel us to try and do something about it. If we see something affecting a particular tree, we may well decide to do something to help it, such as improving soil drainage or removing parasitic growths and so forth, but mostly we just accept trees as they are with all their flaws and idiosyncrasies.

If there is a value to the ideal pattern it is that it can give an orientation to your work. You can use it as a template to focus your work around, but definitely do not view it as something to achieve as a goal.

Ultimately, for me, the concept of structure as identity, relationship and history, the creation of comfort and the relationship of internal and external gravity to structure gives a whole different rationale for the structural work that is well beyond the simple model of ideal gravity lines.

In Fig. 67a and 67b you will see a full pelvis and upper body x-ray of one of my clients. She was 82 years old at the time of the x-ray. I began my work with her the following year. She was bent almost double when walking. She walked with the aid of two walking sticks. She described her spine as looking like a question mark. She was in constant pain. I treated her in her own home. For the first session I worked with her on her bed as she could not get on the portable bodywork table. All I did was work on her water element by stimulating her water finger and toes and connecting them to her water chakra, followed by a 15-minute perineal treatment making connections to her neck and then around the back of her pelvis and lumbar spine. To be honest, considering that the chiropractor she had seen, and who had arranged for the x-ray, had said that the degeneration of the spine was too advanced for him to be able to do any significant work with her, and considering that her medical doctors had indicated that she was beyond any remedial help, and had simply prescribed calcium supplementation and pain killers, my expectations of being able to make any significant difference were not high. Some three days later, when I visited her for the second session, she described how the morning after the first session she awoke without pain for the first time in over three years. By the end of the first 10 sessions, she was able to stand more upright and walk without the aid of the sticks. She had what I would have to call an irascible nature and told me that she had gone to see her medical doctor and, upon walking into the consultation room, had said to him: "Do you want to see a miracle?" She then threw her metal walking sticks into the corner of the room, straightened up and stalked out! I continued working with her for over three years. During that time her mobility improved dramatically and the pain never returned. I never had another x-ray done to see exactly what changes had taken place in the spinal alignment. It was enough for both of us that she was in a place of deep ease and comfort. Her mood and personality underwent considerable change concurrent with the release of the pain and increase in mobility. She was that type of client who, in a certain sense, becomes one of your greatest teachers.

Structural Bodywork

> As a final balancing physical factor, the reaction of the gravity of the earth
> on muscles and joints must not be overlooked.
>
> Vol. I, Book 2, p. 4

In structural bodywork we work from the outside in and the bottom up. In structural sessions we are working back through the layers of compensation to the primary

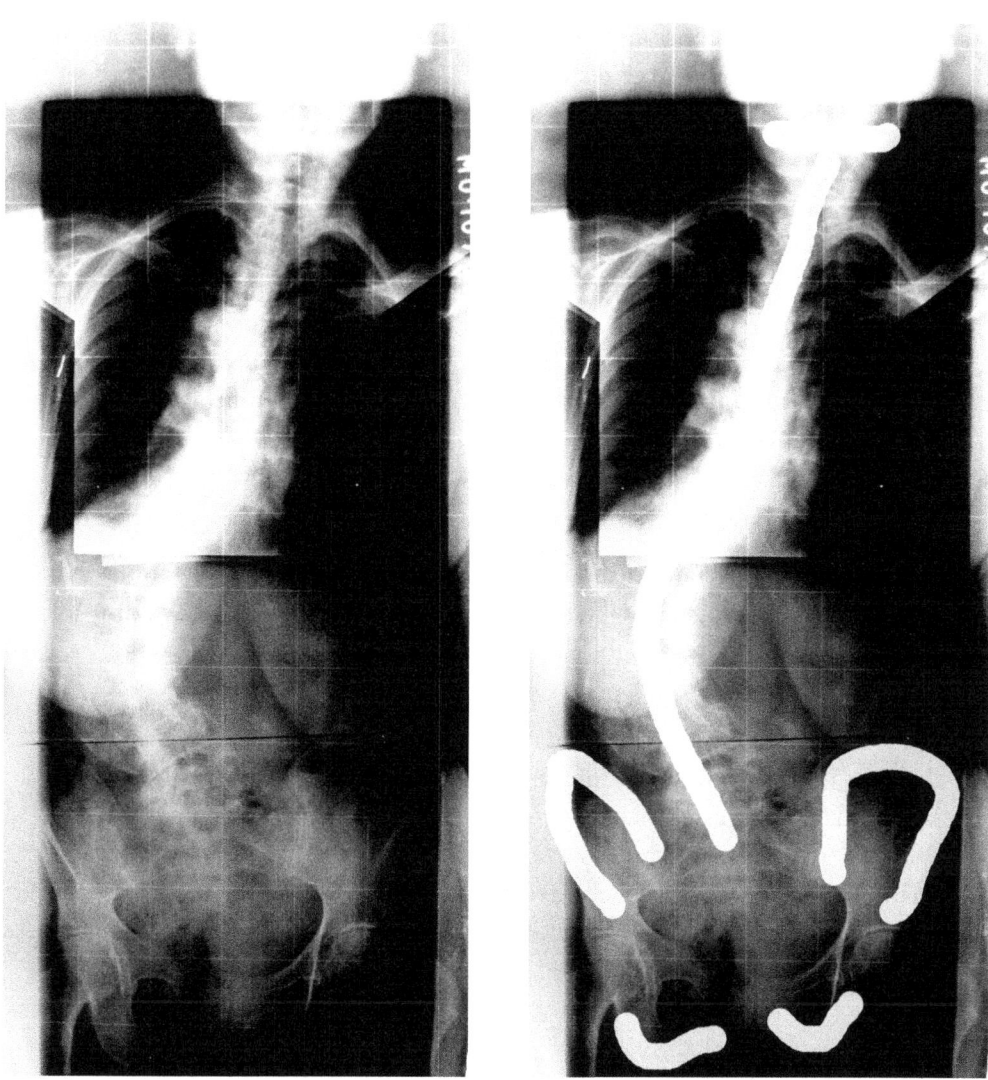

Fig. 67a   **Fig. 67b**

The white shading on the duplicate x-ray on the right is simply to show even more clearly the alignment of the spine and the pelvic position. Even with all the middle and lower body distortion you can see how the cranial base is maintained relatively level. If you have experience in reading x-rays there is much more you can see. This is one of the most extreme distortions of a human structure you are ever likely to see. The fact that I was able to make such a difference to her quality of life is a testament to the effectiveness of the techniques and understanding that Dr. Stone evolved.

adaptation to gravity and then into the forces that underpin the intrinsic alignment to recover a simple elastic and adaptive structure.

A general definition of structural balancing is simply "correcting the bone alignment of the skeleton relative to the force of gravity." As clear as this is, I always wanted a better definition of structural bodywork from a more specific energetic perspective, so I began one of my numerous readings of all Dr. Stone's books. As anyone who has done this will know, the books are far from linear. You can be reading about the colon one minute and on the next page you are into the soul and evolution and then into structure and then to diet. It makes it hard to keep focused on any one topic, as you can veer off and find yourself intrigued by a unique perspective on a different topic and totally lose the thread of your original intention.

However, on reading the small booklet, *The Mysterious Sacrum – The Key to Body Structure and Function*, which is in Volume II, I began to research every reference to the sacrum throughout Stone's writings and realised that the sacrum is the most referenced aspect to structure in all of his writings. The quotes below are unambiguous. I have only added the italics for emphasis, the rest of highlighting is as in the original:

> PHYSICAL BALANCE SUMMARY: The <u>sacrum</u> and the <u>heels</u> have a definite relationship as middle and inferior poles, shown in this chart. When making an examination or a check-up, *see the sacrum as the foundation wedge of support for posture, structure and <u>functional</u> energy impulse.* A brief analysis along these lines will save much time in balancing the structure from the bottom up. In all chronic cases, the root of the trouble is usually hidden here.
>
> Vol. II, Book 5, p. 95

> Tests and *corrections of the sacrum prove its key position in the whole structural economy of the body.*
>
> Vol. I, Book 3, p. 73

> But the sacrum is still the keystone to the royal arch of all structural relation and function in the body's own economy and individual gravity field.
>
> Vol. I, Book 3, p. 72

The sacrum is the vital balancer of the individual energy in relation to gravity. It is the balance wheel of the body's own center of POLARITY, <u>which governs the position of the spinal column</u> through ligamentous and muscular attachments.

Vol. I, Book 3, p. 71

The clearer Polarity definition of structural work is that it is all about sacral balance. So the phrase I was looking for was simply that structural bodywork is "**balancing the three poles of the sacrum.**" The three poles of the sacrum are calcaneus or os calcis, sacrum and occiput. To achieve sacral balance biomechanically means that the head, shoulders and pelvis will need to be level and the spine straight. However, creating an energetic balance of the three poles of the sacrum is conceptually broader than the biomechanical model, and more in line with the creation of comfort. Energetic sacral balance involves creating clear channels of communication and feedback between the three poles.

I also realised that the correction of the os calcis position and the session outlined in charts 54-56 of Volume I, Book 2 (see charts in Fig. 68 below) constitutes a general session for the structure even though the charts only talk about the sequence as a correction for body rotation. The os calcis session actually follows all the requisites of a structural session in that the work is from the bottom up and engages the three poles of the sacrum and *all* the structures in between.

My use of the phrase "general session for the structure" requires a little elaboration before we explore further about the three poles of the sacrum. In its early days,

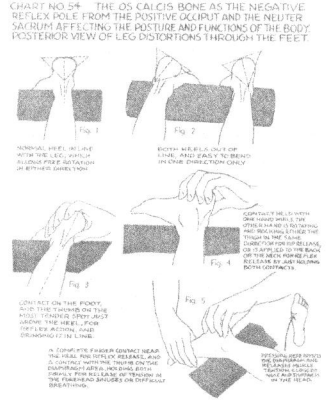 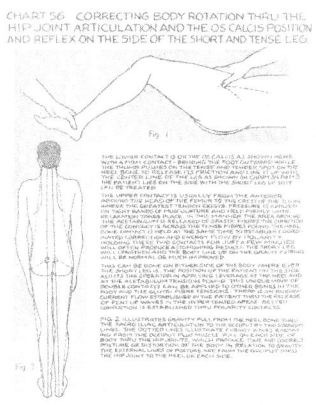 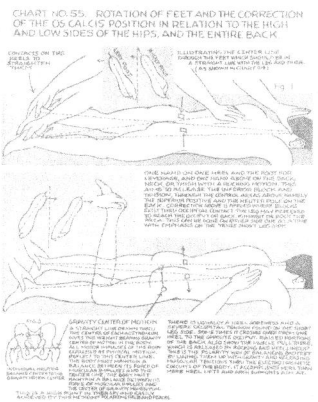

Fig. 68

155

Osteopathy used very specific treatment where such was indicated, combined with a more general treatment approach that over time evolved into a specific segmental approach.

The late British osteopath John Wernham, D.O., a student of Dr. J. Martin Littlejohn, Ph.D., D.O., wrote:

> With the exception of treatment given in the case of acute disease and other certain conditions, osteopathic techniques were always applied under the aegis of the general treatment. There has been a total rebuttal of this first great principle in Osteopathy and operators are content to give only local treatment directed to the painful area indicated by the patient.

> Such a limited viewpoint represents the absolute negation of the second great principle, namely, the integration of all parts of the body, anatomically, mechanically, and physiologically. This is a broad canvas, and if there is detail it must be made to bear a right relationship with the unit body if the condition is to be resolved and the patient stabilised.

> The term "general treatment" fell into disrepute and soon became a background for the so-called 'specific', or 'replacement', techniques which are entirely anatomical in concept and have no concern with the body mechanics, or function. To give a treatment called 'general' gave rise to boredom and led to scant attention to the finer points of our manipulative procedures. It was for these reasons that the old title was abandoned and the new term "body adjustment" substituted.

> The truth is that the general treatment, body adjustment, full treatment, or whatever name is chosen, is the very fabric of our manipulation and demands our closest attention every step of the way.

> The technique employs the long lever and deals with all tissues conjointly, with only special emphasis where it is necessary. The method is deliberately routine in order to ensure that nothing is missed in diagnosis and, further, to establish the lost rhythm so often lacking in the patient. The limb leverage is powerful and brings into play every muscular insertion into the spine and into the pelvis, yet the effect is gentle, smooth and relaxing.

> The objective is the restoration of the internal environment and thus provides those conditions essential for the recovery from the lesion state. Without such preparation, the good effect of spinal correction is limited

and short-lived. In fact, in a great many cases, is the general body adjustment will be enough for nature to make the recovery without any local, or specific, work whatsoever.

But, perhaps, the most important aspect, and the most important argument in support of this traditional technique, is to be found in the long-term effects which are stable and stress-resistant. Finally, it must be said that, although the technique is loosely and freely given, it must be precise and accurate in execution.

Dr. Stone learned both specific and general methodologies in his training between 1910 - 1915. However, in the era he trained in, any health issue presenting as a specific problem was dealt with in a specific way but always in *relation to the whole*.

> Totality is not, as it were, a mere heap [of parts], but the whole is something besides the parts.
>
> *Metaphysics*, by Aristotle Book VIII, 1045a., 8–10

To work specifically and segmentally without regard to the whole is akin to not seeing the forest for the trees or, to use a phrase common in Polarity teaching, "not seeing the Big Picture."

In Polarity, Pierre Pannietier's development of the general energy balancing session was a return to some of the classical principles that Dr. Stone originally learned. So, to have a treatment that is a general treatment for the structure, that addressed it in its totality, was something that intrigued me; and the os calcis session (see p. 210) elegantly fit that definition. However, please don't make the mistake of thinking that the phrase "general session for structure" means it is a generalised approach indicating that you do *exactly* the same thing on each client. The sequencing of manipulations might be the same but the individual tension patterns in the client's body that you address in each phase of the session are always going to be unique.

As Dr. Stone said many times in his books no one pole rules alone; to create true balance in the body all three poles must be worked. The three pole approach of Polarity Therapy is in essence a more integrated and whole body approach to viewing and working with the structure in its totality.

Dr. Stone referred to the sacrum as a "keystone" structure.

> The sacrum is a key wedge between the two innominate bones, like the keystone in an arch, between the two pillars on which this arch rests.
>
> Vol. II, Book 4, p. 6

A keystone is an architectural feature dating back to the Roman era and earlier. The Romans were the first to use arches extensively in their buildings, bridges and aqueducts. The keystone (Fig. 69a) is the wedge-shaped stone placed right at the top of an arch. When building an arch it is the final stone placed and locks the rest of the arch in position.

A feature of an arch with a keystone is that the keystone itself bears very little weight from above because it immediately deflects the vertical weight laterally, and these lateral forces become a kind of thrust or "push" and at the same time a compressive downward force dissipating through the other elements of the arch (Fig. 69b). In the body, something similar to the forces in the keystone arch happens. The innominates (the pelvic bones consisting of both ilia, ischia and pubis) carry the weight of the body, that is, bear the compressive stress, transmitting it down the two pillars of the legs. In a structurally

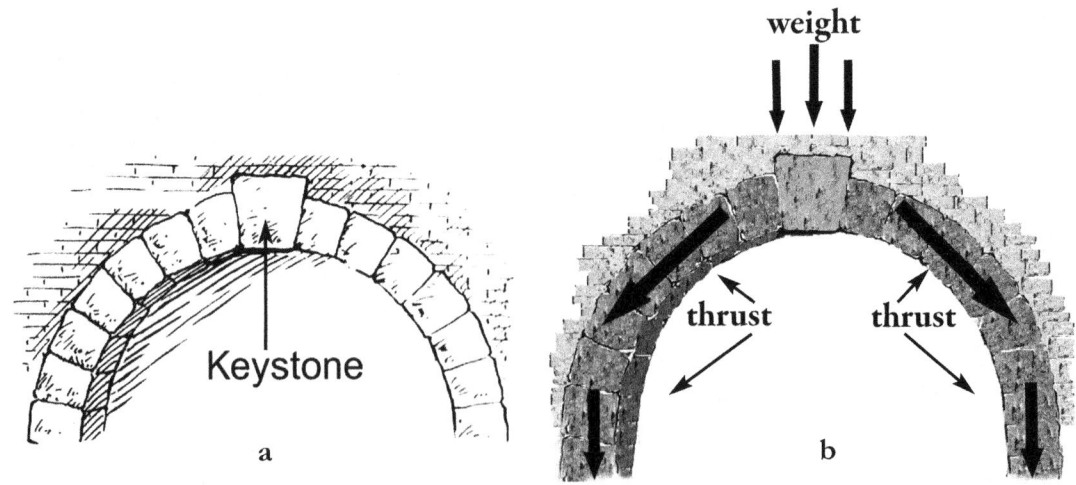

Fig. 69

158

balanced body, the whole weight of the upper body structure is directed downward into the sacrum, which then laterally transmits this force leftward and rightward into the two innominates, and from there down through the legs.

The polarities of the three poles of the sacrum are:

+	Ø	−
Occiput	Sacrum	Calcaneus/Os Calcis

Symmetry of form played a large part in Dr. Stone's concept of the positive and negative poles of the sacrum. The heel, sacrum and occiput have a certain structural symmetry in that they each exhibit a triangular shape. They are all functionally related, being keystone structures in their immediate location, the occiput being a keystone in the vault of the cranium and the heels being the keystones in the arches of the feet.

To create structural balance between these three keystone structures means that there must be minimal energetic, muscular and skeletal issues between the occiput and heels.

Structure and the Elements

Elementally speaking, the structural work, being focused on the skeleton, comes under the classification of earth. It is basically stretch-release, movement and moulding technique. The stretch-to-release aspect makes it functionally similar to the stress positions of Polarity Yoga. Further, just as rocking movement is used in Polarity Yoga, movement in the form of rajasic work is fundamental to good structural bodywork. Rocking motions of two of the three major body masses, the chest and pelvis, are employed extensively, as well as the use of the long levers of the arms and legs to both rock and stretch. The moulding aspect is a basic application of the earth element. Think of a potter moulding clay into a pot or vase, a baker kneading dough, or a child working with Plasticine, modelling clay or play doh. Translate those images into the way tissue is moulded and bone alignment may be altered. I have often said that Polarity's structural bodywork has a deep earthy resonance which reminds me of a slow deep voice like that of Eartha Kitt signing, "The Girl From Ipanema."

A different elemental aspect comes from the pentamirus combinations of the air element, where air represents movement and its interaction with ether and earth, creating two movement variables that are definitely relevant to structural work. When ether modulates the movement of air, there is a *lengthening*, which you could think of as elevation through the structure, an upward movement. When earth modulates the movement of air you get *contraction*, which is not a quality we want to have in excess when dealing with structure. We want a balance of ether and earth, of lengthening and contraction, within the structure.

It is also important to think of the broader resonances of both ether and earth and how the emotional and astrological aspects of these two elements may be playing out in clients' lives and influencing their structures. In relation to ether, it is primarily associated with the emotion of grief and can directly affect the function of the joints in the body. Grief may come from mourning the loss of someone close to oneself, or from any other kind of loss or change, such as in work life or living environment and location. Earth is related to fear and security issues as well as attitudes such as stubbornness, as symbolized by the bull neck of Taurus. Earth also expresses itself as the fear of falling or failing and can affect the knees, which are governed by Capricorn. Internal mental stress caused through the need for life to be perfect can create changes in the bowels, which relates to Virgo. Issues in the colon such as Irritable Bowel Syndrome (IBS) can definitely affect the tension level of the erector spinae of the lower thoracic and lumbar area.

Another elemental consideration is the fact that the sacrum is controlled, in large part, by the water element. The water chakra is located at the lumbo-sacral junction. Any emotional disturbances of a watery nature, such as excessive emotional sensitivity, or addictive behaviour, can directly influence the position of the sacrum. The converse is also true. A sacrum that has moved out of alignment due to compensation or physical injury can cause emotional issues and skin problems.

> The sacrum is the key triangle of the pelvis, registering all the impulses, reactions and disturbances of the watery element in the human body. Especially the skin and mucous functions are affected by the abnormal actions of frustrated impulses and the structural relationship of the sacrum.
>
> Vol. I, Book 3, p. 71

Structure and the Autonomic Nervous System

At the beginning of this chapter I mentioned how important perineal and coccygeal work is to structural balancing. The reason for this is that our posture is not maintained via voluntary control. Posture is an involuntary process. Anyone can alter their posture voluntarily through an act of will. We can stand differently, alter our head position and so forth, but as soon as our attention wanders we go back to our normal, involuntary postural alignment. This involuntary holding is maintained by basal brain structures and through our autonomic nervous system. Thus:

> Rule: No relaxation of the voluntary nervous system can take place as long as the involuntary ones are locked and tense. A bony correction should never be forced. Merely telling a patient to relax is useless. Tension usually goes much deeper than voluntary control.
>
> Vol. I, Book I, pp. 86-87

A more modern term for the voluntary nervous system is "somatic nervous system." The somatic nervous system controls impulses conveyed to the skeletal muscles from the central nervous system. Simply said, the somatic nervous system controls the way in which impulses from consciousness and the brain control the movements of the body. The involuntary nervous system is the autonomic nervous system, consisting of the sympathetic and parasympathetic nerves, which together control all involuntary physiological functions, such as heartbeat, digestion, elimination etc. What Dr. Stone is saying in the quote above is that a person can experience tension in the muscles caused by various life experiences but that, invariably, if it is a long-term stressful stimulus, the tension cannot be released through an act of will because the tension has gone deeper and has become locked into the body by the autonomic nervous system, in particular by the sympathetic branch. The sympathetic nervous system has a great deal to do with the muscular holding patterns in our body due to its control over the fight-or-flight reaction, which requires the mobilisation of muscular energy. It is unfortunate that so many stressful life experiences become coded as dangerous, high level survival issues within the sympathetic nervous system, thereby excessively activating the fight-or-flight response. This response over-stimulates the musculature through the secretion of chemicals that act on vasodilation within the muscles. The sympathetic nervous system also acts through direct nerve innervation, because every skeletal muscle has sympathetic nerve fibres within it as well as somatic nervous system fibres. Dr. Stone always addressed the influence of the autonomic nervous system in relation to the structure:

> Check the body for the over-all picture of the distortion to gravity lines; this may include all three nervous systems in their abnormal functions. And by re-checking, after using the Sympathetic and the Parasympathetic Techniques, through PERINEAL and other POLARITY contacts, it will show how much of this distortion was due to their effects on the skeletal muscles.
>
> Vol. I, Book I, p. 86

And:

> If any distortion has been improved or has disappeared, the cause of it was in the sympathetic and parasympathetic systems' reaction on the skeletal muscles. If structural corrections have taken place, it means that a relaxation in the cerebrospinal system has also been affected.
>
> Vol. I, Book I, p. 89

Use of the perineal and coccyx treatments is fundamental to good structural work. The primary question that comes to mind is which part of the autonomic nervous system to focus on and which of these two treatments to use. There are various ways of deciding, but the way Dr. Stone got around the sometimes thorny and confusing issue of creating the appropriate treatment strategies for working the autonomic nervous system was to work both, activating the parasympathetic and sympathetic nervous systems at the same time. He did this by connecting the perineal floor, which reacts to the parasympathetic branch, to the spinal groove, making contacts over the sympathetic nerve ganglion that lie on either side of the spine (See Vol. II, 25 Charts, Chart 8). Whilst this is completely valid, and an approach I often use, sometimes one needs to be more specific to get the release of the musculature.

When working with hypertonic back muscles, that indicate a high level of sympathetic nervous system involvement, it is tempting to focus on the parasympathetic via perineal contacts to switch off the sympathetic response through parasympathetic activation. My experience is that, in this situation, there is often what Dr. Stone called a "lock" in the nervous system, just as their can be a lock in one of the five elements, meaning that the sympathetic branch is no longer responsive to the overall balancing effect of parasympathetic activation. In this case, we again need to fight fire with fire, meaning the use of coccyx treatment, or "vital pelvic balancing" as Dr. Stone called it, to release the sympathetic nervous system. It can be particularly helpful to combine the coccygeal contacts with contacts to the sympathetic ganglion on either side of the spine. (See Vol. II, Book 5, Chart 14, Fig. 3 and Chart 17, Fig. 3.) This deep activation of the sympathetic branch breaks the lock that is stopping the autonomic nervous system from finding a natural balance. This release allows the smooth interaction of the relaxation and expansion as mediated by the parasympathetic branch with the contraction and activation that is controlled by the sympathetic branch of the autonomic nervous system. The result is a more balanced interaction between these two aspects of the nervous system, with palpable evidence in the associated musculature.

Umbilical Work

Umbilical work can be an important technique in terms of structural work because the umbilicus is very close to the location of the centre of gravity of the physical body. Essentially, when you work on the umbilicus you are balancing the primary polarity of the centre and circumference. On the back of the body it is roughly between lumbar vertebrae 2 and 3. The umbilicus can be connected to virtually anywhere on the body. This technique is usually done by sinking your thumb gently into the navel and then pointing it toward the other contact. It is an extremely useful technique for balancing the function of the major joints of the body. To achieve this, you use a very light sensory type of touch on the joints combined with a directional contact at the umbilicus. You can focus on any joint that is significantly disturbed or balance all the major joints. Dr. Stone showed the umbilicus as a pivotal point at the intersection of the primary lines of force from the pelvis to shoulders that form part of the 5-pointed star.

The Structural Patterns

There are two energy patterns that are fundamental to structural bodywork. They are the 5- and 6-pointed stars. These two patterns are generally understood by most Polarity teachers to be *constructive interference patterns*, taking the term from physics, in that they are created by the interaction of all the primary energy flows in the body. In other words, they have no single source such as a chakra but are created as an effect of the general pulsation of energy throughout the body. Dr. Stone indicated that the four elements are represented in the two patterns as air and earth within the 5-pointed star, and fire and water in the 6-pointed star.

Five-Pointed Star

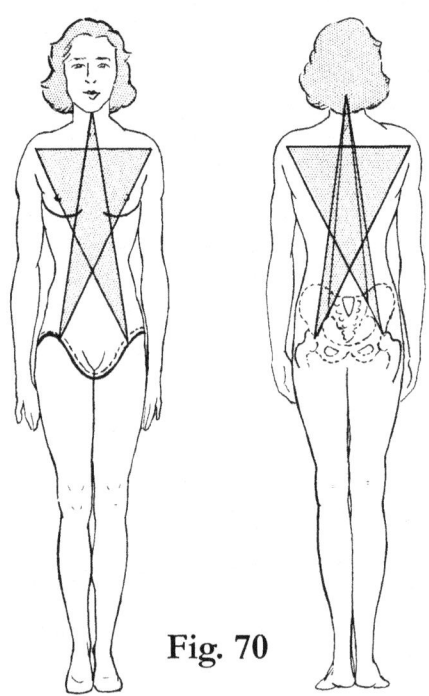

Fig. 70

Historically, Pythagoras taught that the points of the 5-pointed star or pentad relate to the five elements of fire, water, air, earth, and idea. In Polarity "idea" has become Ether. The word Ether is the English version of the ancient Greek word ἰδέα, which actually meant the world of pattern or form. The Pythagoreans also labelled each of the five points of the star with the first letters of the Greek words for each of the five elements which then formed the name of the Greek Goddess of Healing, Hygeia. In Polarity, the 5-pointed star is the symbol of evolution or consciousness rising inwards and upwards from the physical plane back to the causal plane of perfect form and pattern, a return to Source.

In terms of the physical plane and the structure of the body, the pattern relates to the balance of the shoulders and pelvis. In Dr. Stone's charts the pattern is shown as a simple star shape superimposed on the body (Fig. 70). However, in reality it is a more three-dimensional energetic form with multiple lines of force moving both across the body and upwards towards the head. Fig. 71 shows it as multiple lines of force crossing the body, and Fig. 72 gives a better three-dimensional sense of the pattern. A felt sense of the pattern as three-dimensional is essential when using it within the context of structural bodywork.

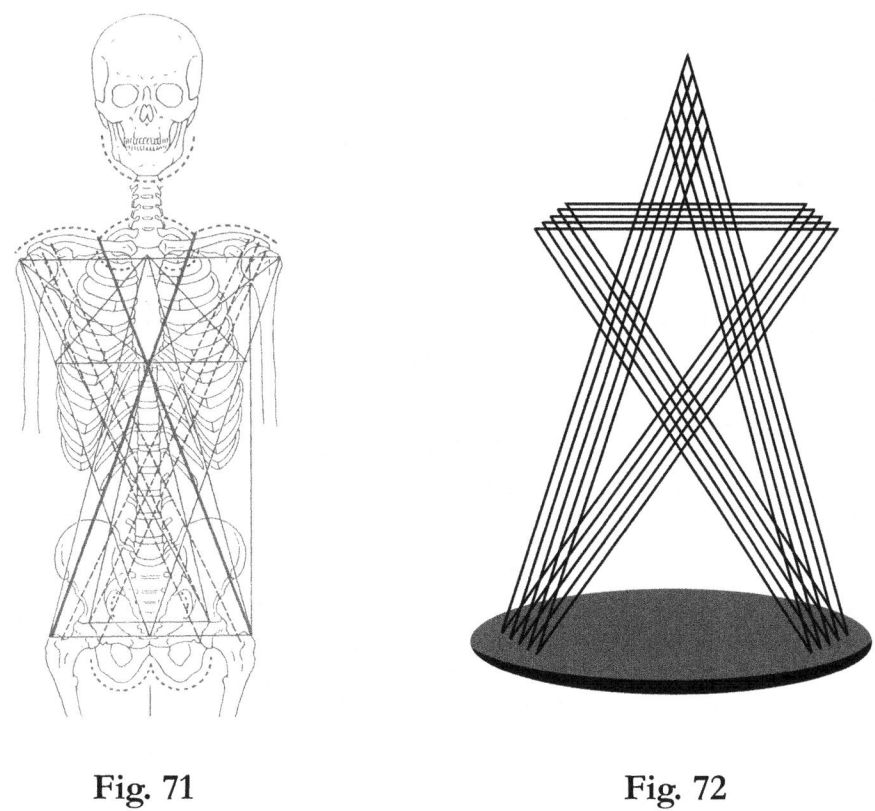

Fig. 71   **Fig. 72**

One can quite easily see distortions of the 5-pointed star in the body. These distortions can range from a collapse of the torso when a person is slumped forward, giving a sense that the star is collapsed, to a contraction on one side of the body where the pelvis is lifted on that side, thereby throwing the base of the star off centre causing the upper part of the star shape to distort. As the 5-pointed star is a structural and energetic pattern, it is not in itself a causative factor in any particular distortion of the star. It distorts due to other changes taking place in the mind, emotions, and energy. These factors affect muscular tension. Another causative factor is simply physical damage to the body. For example, one might have a client who has a strong need to be in control in his or her life, and when experiencing a stressful situation where control is difficult, there occurs an involuntary contraction around the sigmoid valve of this individual's colon. The pain and discomfort of this will affect the position of the pelvis. The primary issue with the valve will cause secondary compensations in terms of muscular balance of the iliopsoas and iliacus muscles on the left side, causing the pelvic basin to shift up and perhaps back on the left, or possibly a lateral translation of the pelvis to the left, or even any number of other combinations of effects. This shift in the pelvic basin in which the lower part of the 5-pointed star sits will cause significant distortion in the lines of force in the star, and this will cause other tertiary compensations elsewhere around the neck and shoulder girdle in the upper part. (See Fig. 73)

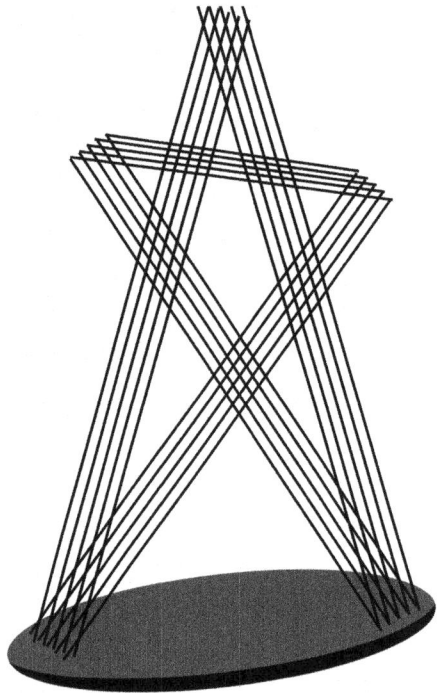

Fig. 73

The benefit of both a visual and a felt sense of the lines of force in the 5-pointed star is the way in which it offers the therapist the possibility of applying corrective stretch release to the body in the appropriate direction.

The fundamental technique for working on the 5-pointed star is shown in Fig. 1 of Fig. 74 (overleaf). It uses directional contacts along the lines of force in the star, working from the pelvis up to the head and diagonally across the body to the opposite shoulder. It can be done on the front and back of the body are the relevant 5-pointed star charts in Volume I, Book 2.

On May 7, 1959 in one of his newsletters, Dr. Stone wrote about this technique. He said:

> Have the patient lie comfortably on his back. With the fingers of both your hands relaxed, place them gently on the inside along the crest of the ilium above Poupart's ligament. Then go deeper, as close to the crest as possible, until you contact the spastic fibers of the iliacus. Hold this pressure firmly for one minute or so, then allow one minute or so for natural reaction and repeat this several times. It is painful and that is why one does not hold the pressure for too long but repeats the process several times. If both sides are spastic, alternate the treatment from one side to the other, several times each; or if only one side is spastic, then treat that side only. This can easily be diagnosed with sensitive touch. As you go deeper and a little superior, you contact the psoas.

As Dr Stone wrote in Fig. 1 of Fig. 74, the key point is the direction of the line of force the therapist applies to the body and energy, "The direction of the arms is toward the opposite shoulder which the operator faces. It affects all the organs above it in that line." And in Fig. 2 of Fig. 74: "A gentle contact first, then steady and specific directional pressure upward until the tissues under the contact relax and reflex that release along the line of force toward the opposite shoulder.

When 5-pointed star work is used on the back of the body, Dr. Stone outlined the technique in sections A and B for Fig. 76 on p. 169. This manoeuvre can done to balance hip and shoulder on the same side when dealing with the pull of gravity straight down, or diagonally when dealing with twists and the effects of reaching upward on one side. Reaching too far in either pulling or pushing actions can trigger reactions in the 5-pointed star. Fig. 75 illustrates the contact points in detail while Fig. 76 shows the hand contacts.

Here are Dr. Stone's explanations and treatments:

CONTACTS ABOVE POUPART'S LIGAMENT TO CARRY IMPULSES ACROSS TO THE OPPOSITE SHOULDER. ILLUSTRATED THERAPY FOR CHARTS 9 AND 10.

THE HAND ILLUSTRATES THE FINGER TIPS MADE EVEN FOR THE CONTACT SO IT HURTS LESS AND GETS AN EVEN PRESSURE ON THE DEEPER MUSCLES.

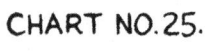

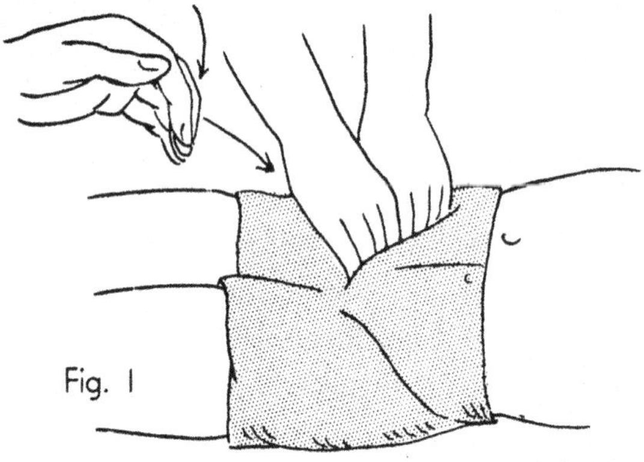

Fig. 1

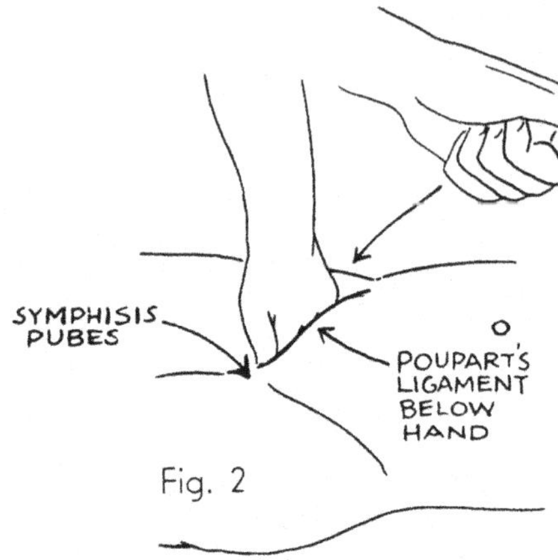

SYMPHISIS PUBES

POUPART'S LIGAMENT BELOW HAND

Fig. 2

A DEEP CONTACT IN THE ILIAC FOSSA JUST ABOVE POUPART'S LIGAMENT. AFTER RELAXING THE SUPERFICIAL ABDOMINAL MUSCLES THE OBJECTIVE IS THE RELEASE OF THE PSOAS MAGNUS AND ILIACUS MUSCLE AND PELVIC BLOCKS. THE DIRECTION OF THE ARMS IS TOWARD THE OPPOSITE SHOULDER WHICH THE OPERATOR FACES. IT AFFECTS ALL THE ORGANS ABOVE IT IN THAT LINE, ESPECIALLY THE STOMACH.

A FIST AND KNUCKLE CONTACT IN THE SAME AREA FOR THE RELEASE OF THE SUPERFICIAL MUSCLES. IT IS GENERAL AND LESS PENETRATING BUT VERY EFFECTIVE IF PROPERLY DONE. A GENTLE CONTACT FIRST, THEN STEADY AND SPECIFIC DIRECTIONAL PRESSURE UPWARD UNTIL THE TISSUES UNDER THE CONTACT RELAX AND REFLEX THAT RELEASE ALONG THE LINE OF FORCE TOWARD THE OPPOSITE SHOULDER.

POUPART'S LIGAMENT

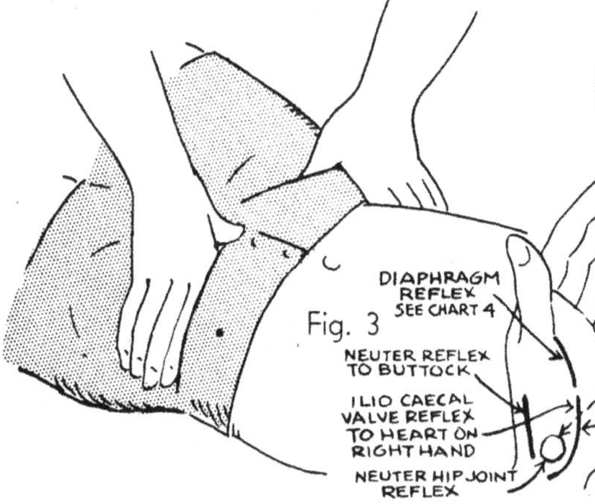

DIAPHRAGM REFLEX SEE CHART 4

Fig. 3

NEUTER REFLEX TO BUTTOCK

ILIO CAECAL VALVE REFLEX TO HEART ON RIGHT HAND

SIGMOID VALVE REFLEX TO HEART ON LEFT HAND

NEUTER HIP JOINT REFLEX

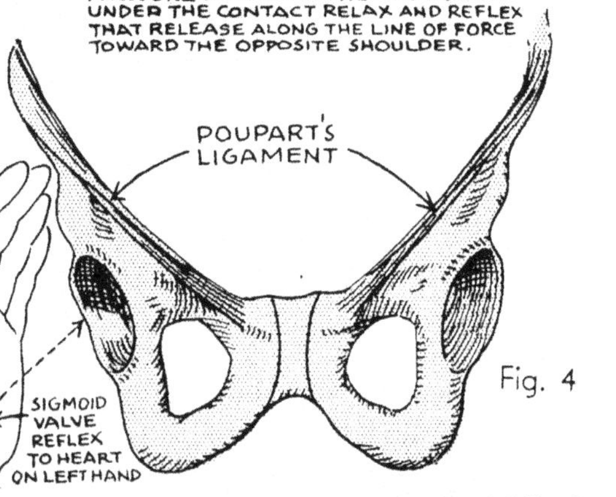

Fig. 4

THE SAME PURPOSE CONTACT MADE WITH THE THUMBS OF BOTH HANDS. THE RIGHT THUMB IS MAKING A SPECIFIC CONTACT ON THE RECTUS ABDOMINALES MUSCLE JUST ABOVE THE PUBIS. THE THUMBS MAKE A SOFTER CONTACT THAN THE FINGER TIPS AND GET A GOOD HOLD ON SURFACE MUSCLES. DIRECTION IS POSTERIOR AND DIAGONALLY SUPERIOR LIKE THE OTHER TWO CONTACTS SHOWN HERE. WHEN THESE AREAS DO NOT RESPOND - FIND THE PERINEAL REFLEX WHICH CONTROLS SPASMS OF INTRA PELVIC MUSCLES AND LEG REFLEXES

A CLEAR PICTURE OF THE ANTERIOR PELVIS AND POUPART'S LIGAMENT TO CLARIFY THE AREA OF CONTACTS ABOVE IT AND ALONG IT'S COURSE FROM THE ANTERIOR SUPERIOR SPINE OF THE ILIUM TO THE SYMPHISIS PUBIS. ANTERIORLY THIS IS THE NEGATIVE POLE TO THE NEUTER DIAPHRAGM AND THE SUPERIOR SHOULDER GIRDLE OF THE TRUNK. THESE GROIN AREAS HAVE A POWERFUL REFLEX AS BASIC AREAS TO THE SUPERIOR DIAGONALLY VIA THE POLARIZED BRAIN CURRENTS OF THE CADUCEUS IN A STRAIGHT LINE THRU THE ELECTRO-MAGNETIC FORCES BLENDING IN WITH GRAVITY.

Fig. 74

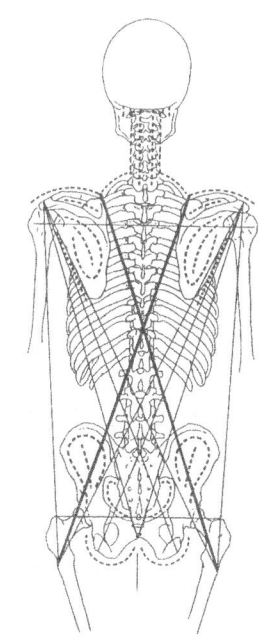

BALANCING
BY CONTOUR

POSTERIOR
GRAVITY LINES

The squares indicate gravity straight downward. The triangles indicate lines of force in motion and stress, in pivoting and reaching. The dotted lines are contact points to balance.

Vol. I, Book 1, Chart 7, p. 78

Fig. 75

A - A firm contact is made with the thumb of the operator on the sorest spot in the gluteus maximum [gluteus maximus] muscle, near its origin, and firmly kneaded; for it is usually congested. If it is too tender, merely hold the contact firmly and gently try different directions of lines of force which release the soreness most, in relation to the muscles of the back.

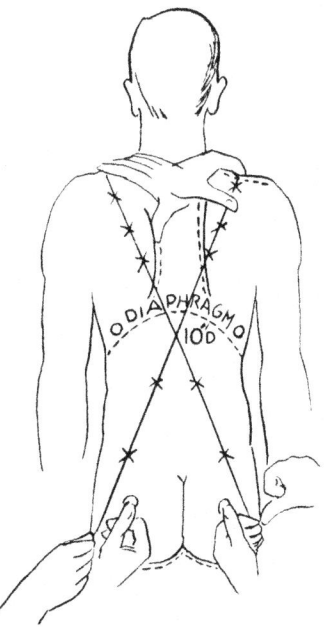

B - A similar contact is simultaneously made on the sorest spot on the shoulder blade, near its spine, and held. That spot is usually very sore. It may be found even on top, near the clavicle or the acromial process [acromion process]. The contact is made on both sides, first one and then the other. Top and bottom on each side correspond, as most of the imposed strain is downward as stationary gravity, in a straight line—not diagonal, as in reaching upward with one arm. But where the diagonal strain is the case, trace it so, and balance it. Hold the sorest spot, which is often the top pole.

Vol. I, Book 1, pp.78-79

Fig. 76

169

Before we finish our exploration of the 5-pointed star, consider Fig. 70 and Fig. 74. A number of geometric shapes, mostly trigons, created by the various lines of force, are visible. These polygons, which relate both to energy and the shape of muscular tissues, have received attention recently in the osteopathic community through the work of Canadian osteopath Robert Johnston. He terms these structures "myogons" in his book, *General Osteopathic Treatment* (Canadian Academy of Osteopathy Press, 2015).

The myogon theory is also related to the common compensatory patterns (Fig. 77) noted by Gordon Zink, D.O. in his 1979 paper "An Osteopathic Structural Examination and Functional Interpretation of the Soma." It is interesting to note that Dr. Stone had seen similar patterns in his work many decades earlier (Fig. 78) and describing them wrote:

> These straight lines are an extension of the brain waves seen as tensions
> with gravity pull in action on muscles of the back.
> Vol. I, Book 2, Chart 7 p. 14

The brain waves Stone is referring to are, of course, the dual descending currents of the ida and pingala or caduceus currents which are the part of the fundamental energy flows that underpin the creation of the 5-pointed star.

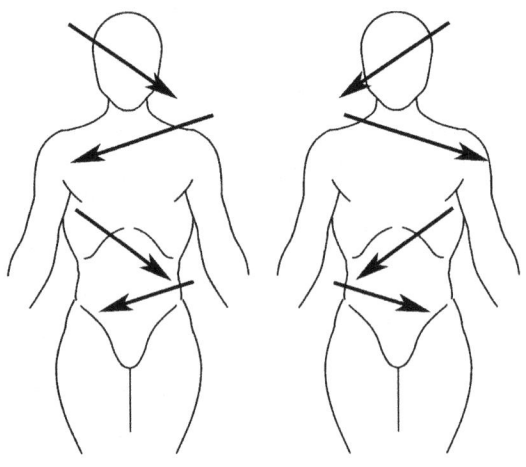
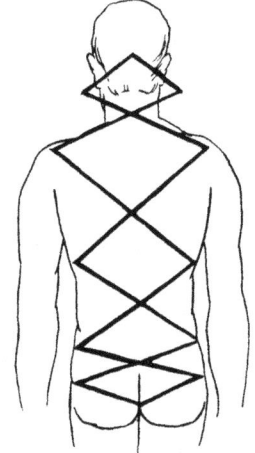

Fig. 77   **Fig. 78**

Six-Pointed Star

Dr. Stone referred to the 6-pointed star symbol as the "The Interfaced Triangles" or the "Seal of Solomon the King." The 6-pointed star has its origin far back in time, appearing both in ancient India and Egypt. As an esoteric symbol, it has many layers of meaning and in a certain sense it is *the* symbol of Polarity Therapy. Dr. Stone also wrote extensively about it in Vol. II, Book 5, Chapter I under the title "The Vital Creative Flame." Dr. Stone wrote that the 6-pointed star symbolises the creation the Jewel in the Lotus Flower of Life:

> This makes the Diamond Soul the perfect product of experience through involution and evolution.
>
> Vol. II, 2 Book 5, p. 9

In one of his lectures in 1960 Dr. Stone said, "The jewel in the lotus; when the shells are cracked then you see the diamond soul which is created by the pressure of the downward current and the pressure of the upward current."

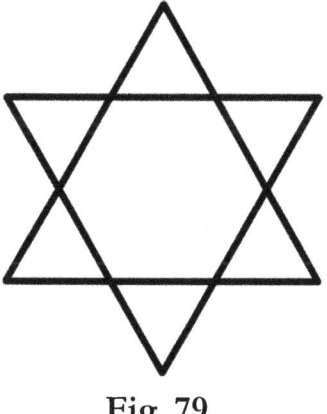

Fig. 79

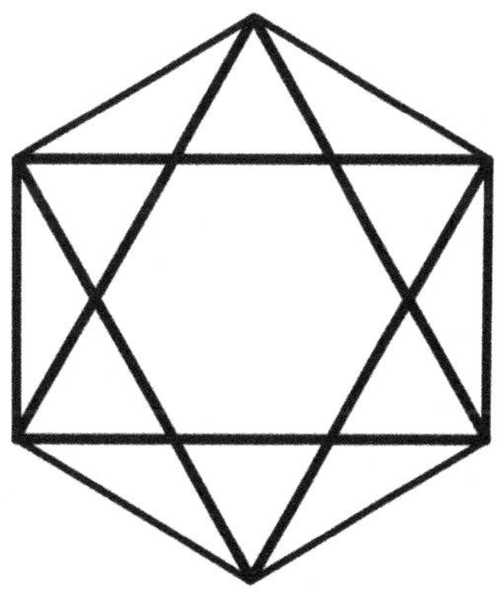

Fig. 80

In Pythagorean teaching, the hexad is called "the form of forms, the articulation of the universe and the maker of the soul." The 6 represents a combination of 1 (energy), 2 (polarity) and 3 (the triad + Ø -); thus 3+2+1=6. The 6-pointed star or interlaced triangles is an innately balanced form that is composed of two triads. By taking a six-pointed star (Fig. 79) and connecting the points of the star, we create the hexagon (Fig. 80) which gives us a key to the qualities of the six-pointed star as structure-function-order. Perhaps the most well-known example of the hexagon in nature is the bees' honeycomb, a natural latticework of hexagons. It is the most efficient, functional use of space and its structure is inherently strong and well-ordered.

Dr. Stone taught that the downward-pointing triangle represents the involutionary process where spirit infuses the material plane, and the upward-pointing triangle is the immediate response in matter that then reaches back up to its source in spirit. It is the symbol of creation. Whilst the pattern could be seen as representing both involution and evolution, overall it is considered to represent the involution of spirit into matter via the creative sexual impulse. This process is union of male and female that manifests a new human life for a soul to express itself through here on Earth.

In Polarity there are many resonances to this symbol: the downward-pointing triangle representing spirit, centrifugal energy, involution, masculinity, individuality or soul essence, fire and extension; and the upward-pointing triangle representing matter, centripetal energy, evolution, femininity, personality, water and compression. Dr. Stone also spoke of the two triangles as being like the gears that must integrate and co-ordinate if the pattern is to balance properly, yet they must also maintain their own uniqueness. In other teachings one will find that some believe the downward-pointing triangle represents the feminine and the upward-pointing triangle the masculine. It is easy to argue it either way, and Dr. Stone would simply say it depends on one's perspective. Is one looking from the Earth up to Spirit or from Spirit down to the Earth? That shift of perspective would change the way one understands what each triangle represents.

Some students and teachers of Polarity Therapy have been confused as to why Dr. Stone drew the interlaced triangles on the back of the body as more compressed than those shown on the front. In his lectures in the 1960s, Dr. Stone mentioned that one could draw the chart differently on both front and back, putting the triangles' bases in different positions thereby, extending the sides and making the form bigger or smaller. In Fig. 81 I have added some dotted lines to a simplified version of his chart in order to make this idea clearer. In a sense, the interlaced triangles are the end points of much larger forms extending up into the heavens as well as down into the Earth.

Calling this particular star pattern interlaced triangles gives a somewhat two-dimensional sense of it, whereas what we are really looking at is a three-dimensional energetic form that is more like two intersecting pyramids (Fig. 82). Fig. 83 shows a three-dimensional shape more akin to Dr. Stone's chart in that the interpenetration of the two forms is such

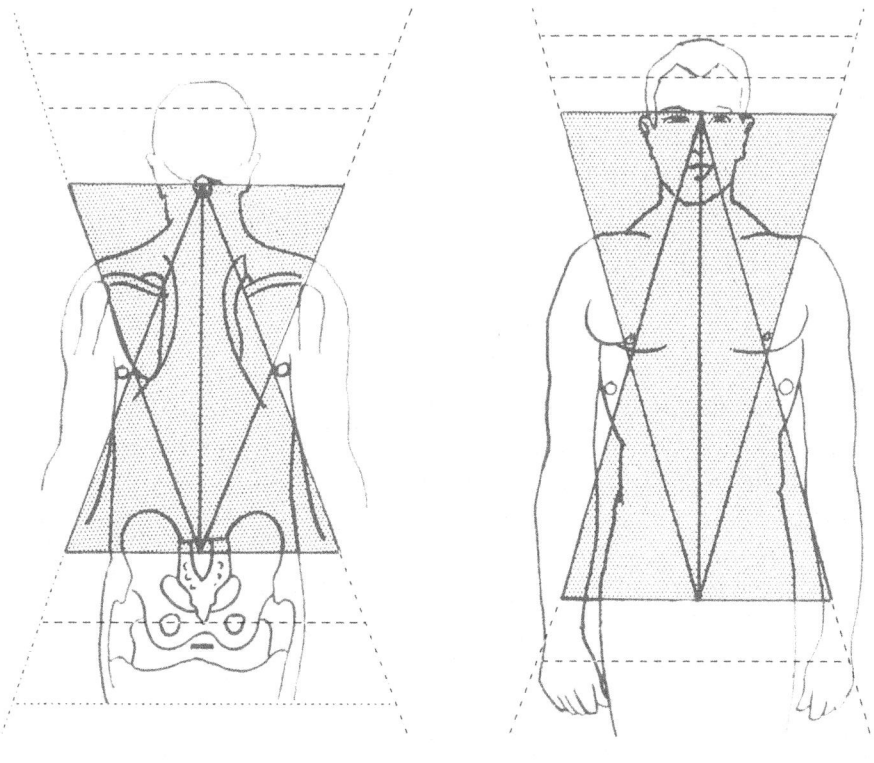

Fig. 81

that bases and apexes almost touch into each other. Fig. 84 shows a deeper interpenetration of the two forms. It is the three-dimensional sense of the 6-pointed star that we need to explore in terms of its influence on body structure.

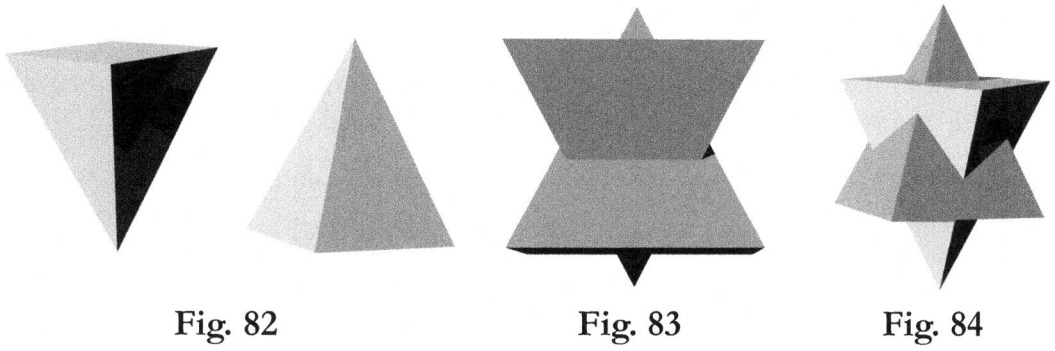

Fig. 82   **Fig. 83**   **Fig. 84**

The fundamental sense of the significance of the 6-pointed star in terms of the structure is the way that the head and the pelvis integrate and balance each other. An image that always comes to my mind is Chinese-style juggling, which is sometimes done with a stick (representing the spine) resting in the centre of the juggler's palm (representing the pelvis), with a plate balanced on top (the head). Any shift in the position of the palm (pelvis) makes an immediate change in the position of the plate (head). This clearly illustrates the influence of a base structure upon other structures higher in the body. Generally, Dr. Stone spoke of the structure as working from the bottom up, referring to the concept by the phrase "as a house rests on its foundation." However, in some people the structure is hung more from the head down than it is built from the bottom up. Actually, the head of an adult is approximately 9% of the body's total weight and therefore can be quite heavy, exerting a substantial effect lower down. Anything that causes a local reaction in the head and neck coupled with a change of its position relative to the centre line, can just as equally influence the position of the spine and pelvis.

Going back to the triad of structure-function-order, we can say that a balanced and integrated 6-pointed star pattern in the human body gives the most efficient usage of physical energy in relation to gravity as well as space for the function of all the internal organs.

In Fig. 85 the black lines represent the downward-pointing pyramid and the grey lines represent the upward-pointing pyramid. Fig. A shows a body with a relatively well-integrated 6-pointed star pattern, though from a purely mechanical perspective its orientation to gravity is a little off centre because the base is not completely parallel to the surface of the Earth. Fig. B shows the way one might visualise the 6-pointed star in a body with very poor posture. There is a complete lack of integration of the two pyramids and an overall disorganisation of both relative to gravity.

In Fig. 86 one can see a rear view of another type of distortion of the 6-pointed star. It is important to remember that, when one senses in three dimensions, one could have a composite distortion that is a combination of those presented in Fig. 85 and 86.

One of Dr. Stone's primary approaches to working with the 6-pointed star, which focused on the pelvis is on p. 229.

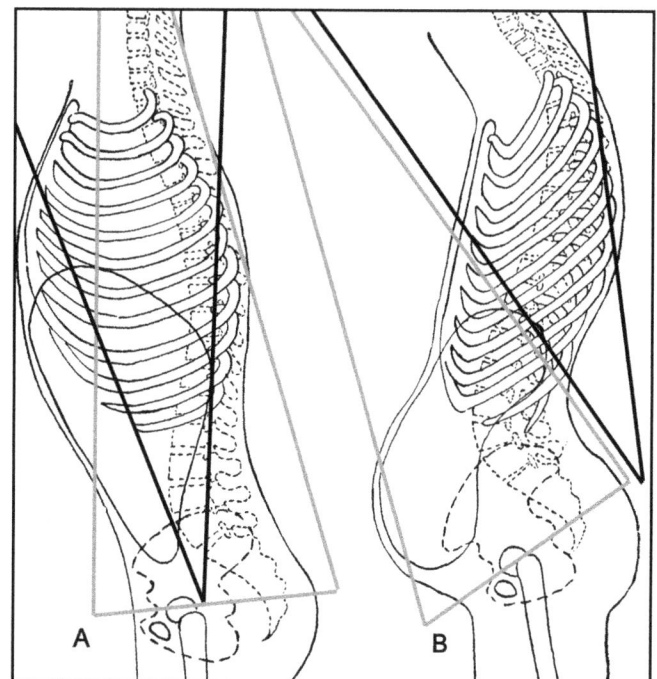

Fig. 85

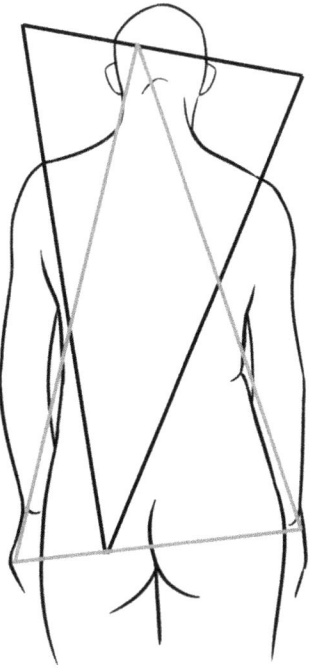

Fig. 86

Treatment

Before exploring treatment theory and strategy I want to outline my basic approach to both the practice and teaching of structural balancing. The first point I want to make is that in no way can structural balancing be taught or practised as a science. By this I mean that the body cannot be assessed and then one decides that the client has a left short leg due to an inferior anterior sacral base on that side or a high left shoulder and a posteriority of the left innominate, and then proceed to treat it by techniques A, B and C. The effects of the techniques are not so predictable, due to the dynamic and individual way each person's body compensates. The approach I use is one of playing with and through the structure of the body, doing a small amount of work and then checking the effect by reading the client again on the gravity board, or by using motion tests, so that I begin to get a sense of the way the client responds to the techniques.

As I explained earlier, a client's sense of identity is often fundamentally related to their structure. It stands to reason that any effective structural session can, in some cases, completely change a person's sense of who they are. This shift can bring up a lot of feelings and the expression of strong emotion. So do be prepared for that possibility.

There are two energy balancing concepts that are intrinsic to structural work. The first is *electromagnetic balancing*, being the simultaneous stimulation of weak areas and sedation of areas of excess energy. Electromagnetic balancing is basic theory in Polarity.

In relation to spinal work, Dr. Stone wrote:

> LOCAL SPINAL ANALYSIS: Every joint is a polarized crossover point for energy waves. The right side is positive (+), the left is negative (-), and the middle is the neuter [neutral] (0) center. The cross-over is bi-polar from the positive right side above to the negative left articulation below it and vice versa.
>
> A sensitive tip of the spinous process is the result of a deep central soreness in the meninges and in the disk [disc]. This should be touched gently with the first finger of the left hand in an upward direction, on the tip of the spinous process.

The corresponding neck vertebra should be held lightly with a double contact with the right hand on the transverse processes, until the soreness lessens.

This is a central core, local balancing of plus (+) and minus (-) impulses. In the last two paragraphs on the next page this local balancing is further explained by tension (which is a minus (-) condition) and by hyperemia (a plus (+) condition), to make it easier to follow.

Vol. II, Book 5, p. 22

Inhibition technique applied in conjunction with electromagnetic balancing is vital in relation to structural bodywork:

First, inhibit the most tender area gently, then more firmly, until this area is relaxed.

Second, use heavy pressure or stimulation on the less tender area, or a constricted area on the spine or back until it lets go.

NOTE: Always remember to use the corresponding POLARITY contact with the other hand. If one contact is heavy, the other should be lighter; if one contact is inhibiting, the other can gently stimulate, depending on the condition and tolerance.

Vol. I, Book I, p. 88

Whilst the quote above relates to perineal treatment, the concepts apply to work on any tight muscles. Chart 22 in Vol. I, Book 2 entitled "Old Moves with New Impetus and Directional Force Applied to Energy Blocks to Release Them" (Fig. 87 overleaf) shows the technique of inhibition applied to tension in the erector spinae muscles.

In modern everyday usage, the word "inhibition" has many shades of meaning having to do with mechanisms of psychological repression. In early Osteopathy, it had a very different meaning. Simply put, when Dr. Stone talked about inhibiting a tension area (a minus or negatively charged area), perhaps in the neck, he meant applying a firm, steady physical pressure, a modulation of tamasic touch. The application of such inhibiting

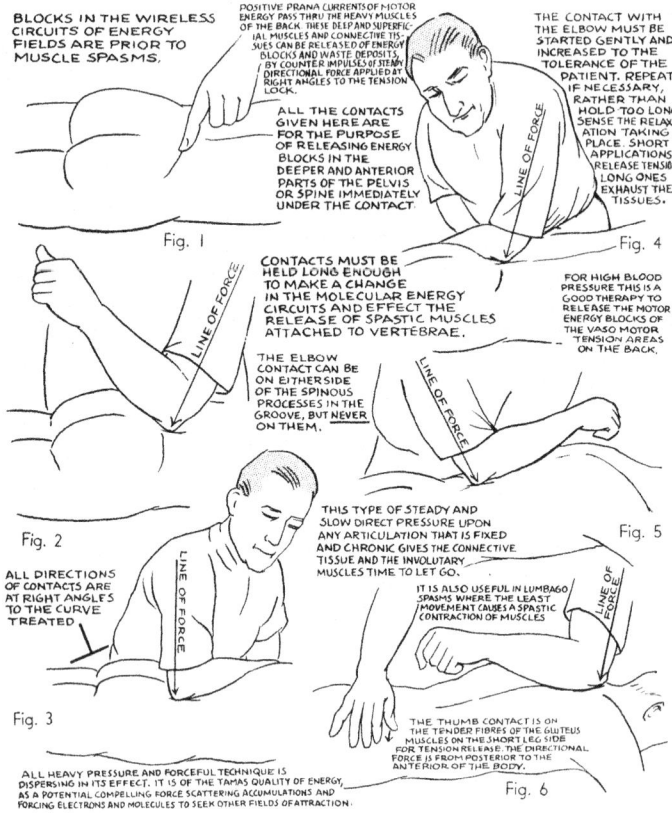

BLOCKS IN THE WIRELESS CIRCUITS OF ENERGY FIELDS ARE PRIOR TO MUSCLE SPASMS.

POSITIVE PRANA CURRENTS OF MOTOR ENERGY PASS THRU THE HEAVY MUSCLES OF THE BACK. THESE DEEP AND SUPERFICIAL MUSCLES AND CONNECTIVE TISSUES CAN BE RELEASED OF ENERGY BLOCKS AND WASTE DEPOSITS, BY COUNTER IMPULSES OF STEADY DIRECTIONAL FORCE APPLIED AT RIGHT ANGLES TO THE TENSION LOCK.

THE CONTACT WITH THE ELBOW MUST BE STARTED GENTLY AND INCREASED TO THE TOLERANCE OF THE PATIENT. REPEAT IF NECESSARY, RATHER THAN HOLD TOO LONG. SENSE THE RELAXATION TAKING PLACE. SHORT APPLICATIONS RELEASE TENSION, LONG ONES EXHAUST THE TISSUES.

ALL THE CONTACTS GIVEN HERE ARE FOR THE PURPOSE OF RELEASING ENERGY BLOCKS IN THE DEEPER AND ANTERIOR PARTS OF THE PELVIS OR SPINE IMMEDIATELY UNDER THE CONTACT.

Fig. 1

Fig. 4

LINE OF FORCE

CONTACTS MUST BE HELD LONG ENOUGH TO MAKE A CHANGE IN THE MOLECULAR ENERGY CIRCUITS AND EFFECT THE RELEASE OF SPASTIC MUSCLES ATTACHED TO VERTEBRAE.

FOR HIGH BLOOD PRESSURE THIS IS A GOOD THERAPY TO RELEASE THE MOTOR ENERGY BLOCKS OF THE VASO MOTOR TENSION AREAS ON THE BACK.

THE ELBOW CONTACT CAN BE ON EITHER SIDE OF THE SPINOUS PROCESSES IN THE GROOVE, BUT NEVER ON THEM.

LINE OF FORCE

LINE OF FORCE

Fig. 2

ALL DIRECTIONS OF CONTACTS ARE AT RIGHT ANGLES TO THE CURVE TREATED

LINE OF FORCE

THIS TYPE OF STEADY AND SLOW DIRECT PRESSURE UPON ANY ARTICULATION THAT IS FIXED AND CHRONIC GIVES THE CONNECTIVE TISSUE AND THE INVOLUNTARY MUSCLES TIME TO LET GO.

Fig. 5

IT IS ALSO USEFUL IN LUMBAGO SPASMS WHERE THE LEAST MOVEMENT CAUSES A SPASTIC CONTRACTION OF MUSCLES

LINE OF FORCE

Fig. 3

THE THUMB CONTACT IS ON THE TENDER FIBRES OF THE GLUTEUS MUSCLES ON THE SHORT LEG SIDE FOR TENSION RELEASE. THE DIRECTIONAL FORCE IS FROM POSTERIOR TO THE ANTERIOR OF THE BODY.

Fig. 6

ALL HEAVY PRESSURE AND FORCEFUL TECHNIQUE IS DISPERSING IN ITS EFFECT. IT IS OF THE TAMAS QUALITY OF ENERGY, AS A POTENTIAL COMPELLING FORCE SCATTERING ACCUMULATIONS AND FORCING ELECTRONS AND MOLECULES TO SEEK OTHER FIELDS OF ATTRACTION.

Fig. 87

pressure, particularly when applied to areas beside the vertebral bodies where the sympathetic nerve ganglion lie, is done to affect the vasodilation/vasoconstriction in that area. In general, inhibition creates vasodilation which brings more arterial blood to the area and more fresh prana. In contrast, particularly if it is being used rajasically to stimulate the opposing area, inhibiting pressure will actually sedate that area through increasing the vasoconstriction and limiting the energy supply, which is the opposite of what one might expect!

The use of inhibition to influence the movement of blood and energy is to use the power of tamas to clear old stagnant blood and energy from an area in the body. Inhibition is a level of pressure that does not take a client too far beyond their comfort zone. It challenges but does not damage the tissues you are working on. Inhibition technique is, in essence, high quality deep tissue work. It should not be confused with the still rather too prevalent interpretation of tamasic bodywork in Polarity, which can only be called deep pressure work in which the practitioner presses as hard as possible on the client's body. (It may be beneficial at this point to re-read Chapter One for my deeper discussion of the qualities of touch.)

The second fundamental concept in structural balancing is *balancing by contour*. In his first book, Dr. Stone referred to balancing by contour a number of times. It is his re-statement and application of the concept known as the "Doctrine of Signatures." I have often referred to this as *symmetry of form*. Very simply, it means that any structure in the body has an energetic resonance or correspondence to other structures of similar contour, shape or form. Dr. Stone often used this concept to establish the opposite polarities for any particular part of the body. He used it to discover the positive and negative poles of the triangular sacrum where the similar triangular shape of the os calcis and occiput is the indicative factor. Balancing by contour is a major key to understanding many of the more obscure body relationships that Dr. Stone used in his work.

Historically, balancing by contour has perhaps been most used in herbalism as a way of understanding the healing properties of any particular herb. The concept dates back to ancient Greece. It was used by Paracelsus who wrote:

> Nature marks each growth… according to its curative benefit.

The concept was probably first discussed in detail by Jacob Boheme in 1621 in his book 'SIGNATURA RERUM; THE SIGNATURE OF ALL THINGS. Shewing the Sign and SIGNIFICATION of The several Forms and Shapes in the Creation AND WHAT THE BEGINNING, RUIN, AND CURE OF EVERYTHING IS.' In his book Boheme wrote:

> Thus everything which is generated out of the internal has its signature; the superior form, which is chief in the spirit of the working in the power, does most especially sign the body, and the other forms hang to it; as it is to be seen in all living creatures, in the shape and form of the body, and in the behaviour and deportment, also in the sound, voice, and speech; and likewise in trees and herbs, in stones and metals; all according as the wrestling is in the power of the spirit, so is the figure of the body represented, and so likewise is its will, so long as it so boils in the life-spirit.

Dr. Stone wrote:

> Hence all construction must start first with designs of blueprints and patterns of things to be created, built or made. As the pattern is, so is the structure in its relation and function to all parts as a unit. Geometry and geometric proportions are the first process of creation in the great and in the small. 'God geometrizes.'
>
> Vol. II, Book 4, p. 51

One of the many examples of its use in structural bodywork is when Dr. Stone wrote:

> The very shape of the ear shows POLARITY association with the similarly formed innominate
>
> Vol. I, Book 3, p. 49

This is shown in the technique for "Innominate, Temporal and Occipital Release" in Vol. I, Book 3, Chart No. 16 and in this book on p. 238. He further writes:

> This treatment is definitely indicated in all cases of ear trouble as well as hip pain, distortions and posteriorities. It POLARIZES AND RELEASES both regions for further correction.
>
> Vol. I, Book 3, p. 49

All drawn from the idea of balancing by contour and the symmetry of form or resonance between the shape of the ear and that of the ilium.

Connective Tissue

> In the structural field of anatomy, it is the connective tissue which is the tension factor for postural relationship and balance response, or the structural lesions in articulations and joints. Posture depends on this relationship of electromagnetic tension fields in the body structure and functional response through the life-breath, the prana currents.
>
> Dr. Stone. *1970 Notes and Findings - Energy Tracing,* p. 7

Working with the fascia is an important part of structural work. I have explored Dr. Stone's thoughts on connective tissue in the book, *Pranotherapy - The Evolution of Polarity Therapy and European Neuromuscular Technique.*[1]

Body Reading

Before approaching any form of structural body work one needs to have a clear picture of the client's structure. To do this requires the development of the skill of body reading. When I think of the whole process of body reading, a phrase that comes to my mind is *the total bodily gesture in space.* If you consider how, whilst visiting a museum or art gallery, you take in a sculpture, you would, in all probability, walk around it, perhaps even crouching down so as to be able to see it from many different angles so you could achieve a total appreciation of it. If you think of the body as a living sculpture the same ideas apply. You are looking for a three-dimensional experience of the client's body. In the standard gravity board body reading outlined by Dr. Stone, the practitioner primarily focuses on the rear view of the body. This is important but other perspectives are equally so. In this regard:

> Merely measuring man's relationship to gravity is not sufficient.
>
> The line-up has been used in this manner for a long time and it has been found wanting because the relationship of a living being is quite different than an inert mass. The purely mechanical principles do not suffice here. After many years of checking and using this simple device, I stumbled onto the idea how this could be used in measuring the POLARITY FIELDS OF THE BODY AND CHECKING THEIR RELATIONSHIP WITH EACH OTHER against the background of the earth's gravity.
>
> Vol. I, Book 3, pp. 63-64

There are three basic types of body reading. The first is when the body is lying down and the second and third are when standing. In the first type, gravity is not a major influence, whereas in the other two it is the primary factor. When a client is lying on the table, the effect of gravity is largely neutralised. Body reading done when the effect of gravity is reduced tells you about the client's relationship with their inner life. You are seeing a

---

1. By Phil Young, Dr. Randolph Stone and Dewanchand Varma, Published by Masterworks International, 2011

person's internal relationships to and between their mental and emotional centres of gravity. Please refer back to Chapter 3, p. 33 for more detail on this type of body reading.

Of the two types of body reading done when standing, where gravity is the primary factor, the side view is done to evaluate the energy levels in the five elements as expressed through the position of the spine and oval fields. The rear view, which will be explored in greater depth later in this chapter, tells about a client's relationship with their outer life, that is, how the client deals with external forces and personal relationships.

Simply reading the body in relation to gravity tells a great deal about structural distortions and the body's ability to adapt to stress but tells little about the status of the internal physiological and energetic functions. That requires integration of information gained from using all three types of body reading, standing (rear and side view) as well as lying down.

The use and training of the visual sense is crucial to being able to read the structure. It is also valuable to develop the ability to use the kinaesthetic sense to mirror a client's structure, a process I call *postural mirroring*. In essence, one must train one's own body to mimic the client's structure in order to sense the dynamics involved in the client's posture. This kinaesthetic mirroring technique conveys an enormous amount of information about the stresses and strains in the client's body. Essentially, this mimicry places similar strains momentarily on one's own body. Like any technique, the more one practices postural mirroring, the better at it one becomes. I suggest doing this with all clients for some time before beginning to use the gravity board to get the "feel" of your client's structural patterns.

The Side View

The side view of a client is important because it tells which of the elements are energetically activated and which are depleted. The cervical spine indicates the activity of the ether energy, the thoracic spine the activity of the air energy, the lumbar spine the activity of the fire energy, and the position of the pelvis indicates what is happening in the water and earth energies. If there is a significant depletion in any element, the therapist needs to rebuild that lost energy because none of the structural corrections will hold if there is an underlying weakness in any energetic element, particularly in those elements directly linked to a spinal level that may be the focus of attention in the work on the structure.

The simple sketches in the illustrations below and overleaf convey a sense of what will be observed when the structure at a particular spinal level is either activated or depleted.

Ether

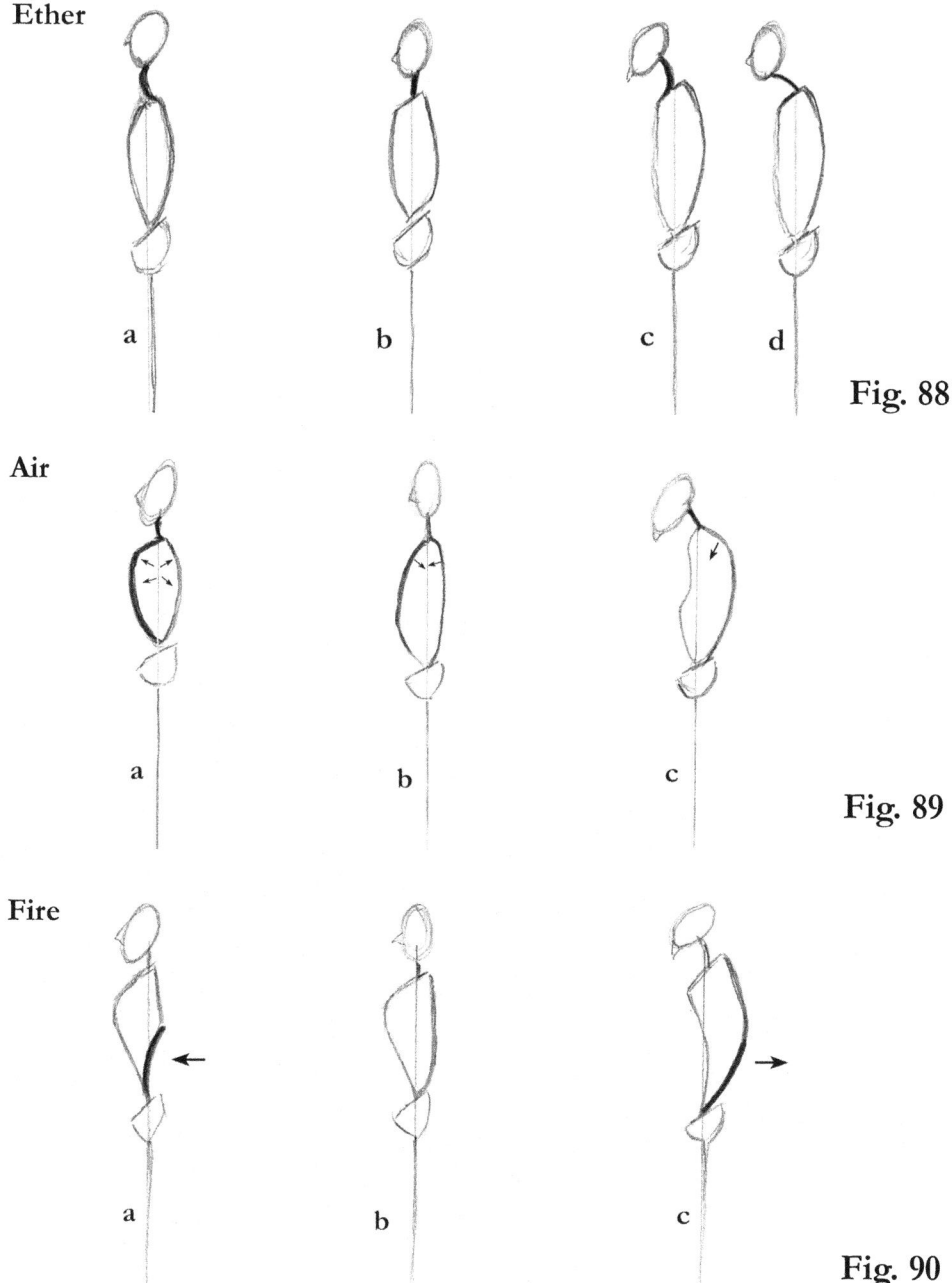

a   b   c   d

Fig. 88

Air

a   b   c

Fig. 89

Fire

a   b   c

Fig. 90

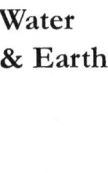
**Water
& Earth**

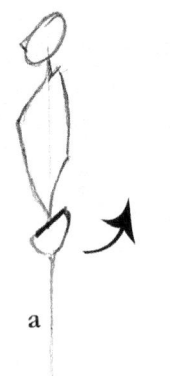
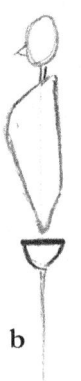
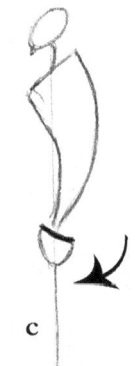

a   b   c

Fig. 91

Element	Part of Spine	Energy Activated	Energy Depleted	Fig. no.
Ether	Cervical	Lordotic curve, nose up slightly	Straight, kyphotic curve or collapsed forward (head butting)	Fig. 88
Air	Thoracic	Kyphotic curve and gentle lift at the sternum	Collapsed at front (hollow), straight thoracic spine, generally deflated (like a collapsing balloon)	Fig. 89
Fire	Lumbar	Lordotic curve	Straight or kyphotic curve	Fig. 90
Water & Earth	Pelvic	Tilted gently forward at iliac crest, tail lifted	Tilted back at iliac crest, tail tucked under	Fig. 91

Illustration "a" in each sketch shows the element and its related spinal segment with an optimal level of energy. Illustration "b" in each sketch indicates a transitional stage wherein energy is either building or becoming depleted. Illustration "c" (and "d" in Fig. 88) indicates a significant depletion of energy.

The table opposite outlines the way in which the spine is affected in respect to the side view when the energy is either active or depleted.

There is a more complex reading of the structure in relation to the mindset and play of emotions within each element as the structure shifts from activation through transition to depletion that is usually referred to as the 'Energy Stress Model.' Readers wishing to know more about the Energy Stress Model are invited to read the forthcoming book, *Self-Defence Strategies* by Morag Campbell and Phil Young, Masterworks International, 2017.

Rear View - The Gravity Board

The rear-view body reading that Stone used as his primary tool to evaluate a client's structure was done on the gravity board. This device uses a plumb line as the guide to the way a body should organize itself in relation to gravity if it is to be considered to be economically working with that force rather than against it. The plumb line is also the "mirror" that shows precisely how the body is deforming in relation to gravity. When a client is standing on the gravity board, the distortions of the skeletal frame caused by unequal muscular tensions become visible.

The gravity board[1] itself is made of a wood and is 24 inches long by 12 inches wide (61 cm. x 30.5 cm.). It has a central wooden divider that is 2½ inches (6.35 cm.) wide and one inch (2.5 cm.) high. This divider should have a line drawn along its full length which is in the exact centre line. The cross piece or backstop is 1 inch (2.5 cm.) wide and 2 inches (5 cm.) high. There should be a small spring affixed to one end of the divider to which is attached the plumb line when using the board. The spring is used because a freely hanging plumb bob moves about far too easily. A plumb bob is necessary in order to establish the correct alignment of board and string. Later, for speed of setting up, the board should always be placed in the same position on the floor and the plumb line hung from the same spot on the ceiling. This can be done by marking the place on the floor where the board is to be situated, so that it is not necessary to re-check its position in relation to the plumb line every time it is used. It is also possible to do as Dr. Stone recommends and have the

1. Visit http://www.masterworksinternational.com/polarity/gravity-board for detailed instructions on making a gravity board.

board close to a wall with long hinges attached to it, so that when it is not in use it can simply be moved up out of the way. Dr. Stone modified the design of the board over a number of years. Primarily, he widened the distance between the feet. For ease of set-up, a permanently fixed board is most desirable.

Dr. Stone explains the value of the plumb line:

> THE PLUMB LINE is at least as old as the pyramids. The plumb line indicates the relationship of a horizontal base - representing the earth or foundation - to the upright line of force as the supporting beam from north to south - head to feet - as the shortest line of gravity pull. For checking the body's muscular contractions in relation to gravity by the plumb line method, the feet are placed in a square angle like a cross, and the plumb line should be in line with the center part of the board. Then minor deviations of angles and joints are clearly discernible against this background of a central line in perfect relation to the gravity pull.
>
> Vol. I, Book 3, p. 19

To see all of the distortions in the client's structure, the client should be fully undressed whilst on the gravity board. Figures in this book reflect that protocol. However, there are a great many issues that can arise in asking a client to fully undress. Most people experience considerable discomfort at the idea of another person staring at their naked body even if it is from the back. Be sensitive to the emotional issues of the person on the gravity board. Remember they are in a vulnerable state of mind. If someone has a problem undressing for the gravity board reading, make sure to get a clear description of the exact nature of the problem they have with the process because only then can there be a sensitive solution. There are various strategies to facilitate the body-reading process, ranging from suggesting the person wear a one- or two-piece swimsuit or leotard to simply wearing close-fitting clothing. With some clients, it is worth beginning with them being fully clothed whilst on the gravity board, because even then it is possible to get useful, although more general, information from a clothed reading. Sometimes, after an initial experience clothed, a client may later offer the possibility of reducing the amount of clothing so that more specific information can be gained.

I recommend that any Polarity practitioner about to learn or beginning to explore the use of structural work in their practice start by doing a structural body reading before and after *all* their Polarity sessions. This body reading should go on long before beginning any actual structural bodywork. Body reading practice helps the practitioner get a *feeling* for body reading and the information it can provide and how it can be applied to hands-on practice, so that the he or she is well prepared before beginning to do full structural sessions. Furthermore, one of the major benefits of doing this is so that the practitioner learns that he or she is always affecting structural change even when not precisely focusing on the structure because, as explained earlier, the movement of energy has a powerful influence on structure. It does not matter whether one is simply doing some form of general energy balancing, interacting deeply with the five elements, using nervous system technique or doing reflex work, the structure will respond. It responds because any of this work can and will influence some of the feedback loops between energy, structure and function and because of shifts in a client's internal centres of gravity and sense of self. I should point out that if one does not notice any structural change it is probably because there are so many layers of compensation in the body that it has lost all its elasticity and can no longer respond to more general energy work. In this case the practitioner will need to use specifically-focused structural work in order to affect change.

One thing I quickly learned when doing a body reading on the gravity board is that clients lose sight of the plumb line! I have lost count of the number of times I have had a client walk straight into the plumb line knocking it aside as they got on the board. Now my basic strategy is to place one foot on the board and to curve my hand around the plumb line as I invite them to stand on the board. When I do that, I have yet to have a client walk into my hand or kick the board.

> A right angle is the shortest line to the earth in its gravity pull. The plumb bob test string represents this line. The patient is placed with the back toward this line for comparison and check of the central axis of his own gravity to that of the earth. By doing this, the comparison reveals the imbalance of the person's own gravity structure. This imbalance limits his motion and function, even though he is not in action or under the pull of gravity outside.
>
> Vol. I, Book 3, pp. 63-64

The client stands on the front half of the board so that the heels fit snugly into the backstop of the central divider on the board. In relation to this Dr. Stone wrote:

...and the feet in a natural position, without any effort to place them or line them up with the center of the board. The knees must be free. If they interfere, then the feet should be separated but at an equal distance from the center on each side of the divider, and the heels remaining snug against the back stop.

Vol. I. Book 3, p. 63

This might involve having a couple of extra pieces of wood placed on either side of the gravity board to widen it so that the client's feet remain flat and comfortable. The client is instructed to focus eyes on a point on the wall opposite, at eye level, as this helps to prevent undue swaying of the body. The practitioner sits behind the client and takes a line of sight which always keeps the plumb line aligned with the centre line of the board.

When looking at a client on the gravity board, I begin my reading from the bottom up, beginning with the heels and legs, then checking the "c" line beneath the buttocks. I then check to see whether the plumb line falls directly between the crease in the buttocks. If it falls either to the left or the right it indicates a body rotation backward on that side. I also look to see if there is any deviation of the very top part of the buttock crease. Sometimes it can point slightly to the left or right, indicating that the sacral base is low on the side it points towards. I then check the "b" line for the hip level. At this point I look at the spinal alignment against the plumb line to see whether there is any scoliosis or curvature and note this. I note any skin folds in the waist area caused by contracted muscle groupings on one side or the other. Finally, I note the high shoulder, indicated by the "a" line, the scapula position by looking at the bone structure and shoulder crease at the armpit because this is another useful indicator of shoulder height. I note the position of the arms relative to the side of the torso, noting any differences left to right, and lastly the orientation of the head. I also want to note whether there is any overtly emotional statement being made by the back of the body. As an example, you can sometimes look at the back of the body and immediately see/sense anger or resignation.

Having studied their positioning for a few moments to gain an overall sense of their structural relationship, Dr. Stone suggests that the practitioner take a skin pencil or make-up pen and mark any tense muscles which are bulging towards you with a plus sign and any hollow areas with a minus sign. This is important because, when the client lies down, the tension patterns are often changed or reversed. These marks are a reminder as to

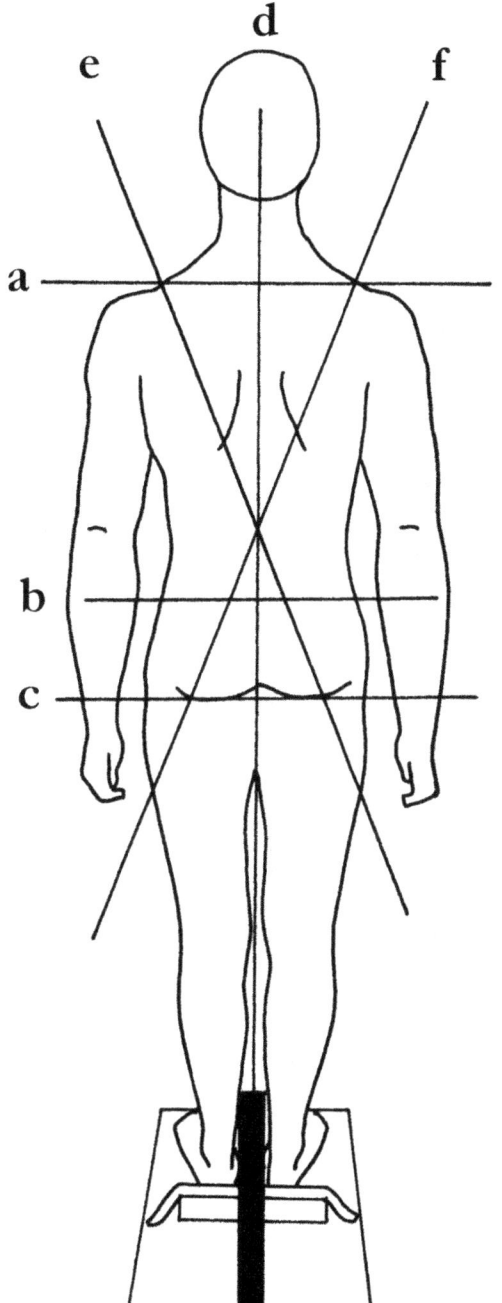

Fig. 92

Body with Perfect Gravity Lines

In the Fig. 92 opposite you will see a body that is lining up perfectly with gravity. The upper horizontal line marked "a" shows level shoulders. The horizontal line marked "b" shows level innominate bones. The horizontal line marked "c" shows a level sacral base. The central vertical line (the plumb line) marked "d" shows a perfectly straight spine with no rotation. Note also that the shoulder blades are level and that there are no skin folds showing in the waist area. The lines marked "e" and "f" are diagonal or a five-pointed star relationship of lines of stress that pass "f" from the hips through the sacro-iliac articulations to the middle points of each shoulder. These two lines cross between the second and third lumbar vertebrae which is at the same level as the umbilicus. Dr. Stone points out that this is the centre of gravity in the body. From the biomechanical perspective this is an ideal body pattern.

where one needs to work. These areas marked plus and minus can be polarized with one other or to the centre of gravity of the body.

As I said earlier, the key to structural work is the position and balance of the sacrum and so a large part of reading the body on the gravity board is to understand the position of the sacrum. To that end there a set of a sacral indicators, certain alignments that give clues as to the position of the sacrum. When talking about the sacrum, the language Dr. Stone used to describe its position focused on the sacral base. The sacral base can be anterior-inferior on one side, the other side being posterior-superior. In other words, the sacral base on one side is low and forward relative to the other side which is high and backward. We are actually talking about very small movements; just a few millimetres or fractions of an inch.

The Sacral Indicators

An anterior-inferior sacral base side is indicated by the majority of the following being on one particular side of the body when viewing the client on the gravity board:

- Low shoulder

- High iliac crest (low ischial tuberosity)

- Low buttock (for this reading to be valid the buttock muscles must have good tone)

- Anterior side of the body (gluteal tension on opposite side)

- Gluteal crease direction points to inferior side

- Occipital tension and mastoid pain is on the opposite side to the inferior sacral base

Other related body readings that can indicate the anterior sacral base side are:

- Skin folding: This is not a definitive indicator. The skin folding is caused by a contraction of the tissues on either side of the spine and is usually related to the high iliac crest and low shoulder on the anterior-inferior sacral base side. However, curvature of the lumbar and thoracic spine to the anterior-inferior sacral base side can create a skin fold on the opposite side of the body. You should correlate the skin folding with other sacral indicators.

- The short leg: Whilst an important indicator, it is not definitive because there can be multiple compensations affecting leg length, and things as simple as man-made clothing can influence the short-leg reading as such material can interfere with the surface energy current flow.

Dr. Stone wrote of the relationship between the short leg and sacral position:

> The shorter of the two legs, according to therapeutic measurement, relates mostly to the electromagnetic central-core over-all stress of the individual through the sacrum and the foramen magnum, by internal muscular tension. Structurally, an anterior sacral base is the cause of the short leg, and not a posterior innominate as was usually taught.
>
> Vol. I, Book 3, p. 71

So, if the client has a low left shoulder, high left hip, low left buttock, gluteal crease pointing to the left and skin fold on the left side as well as a left short leg and soreness over the right side of the occiput/mastoid area then you can be almost certain that they have a left inferior anterior sacral base.

However, as Dr. Stone, wrote:

> Of course, any distortion or abnormality is possible, but those mentioned here are common among the regular run of patients.
>
> Vol. II, Book 4, p. 19

Structural Ideograms

When reading a client's body, I normally make a simple diagrammatic sketch of my findings as I go along. The reader should learn how to draw a small body map of the specific structural readings that are seen. This is not a complicated process and does not require any artistic skill. For example, drawing two short lines one, slightly higher than the other, could indicate a high pelvic crest on one side. A curved arrow can indicate body rotation. A sloping line can show relative shoulder heights. An L-shaped line can show the scapula position. A simple, appropriately curved line indicating the spinal curvature seen from the back, topped by a horizontal line for the head position, can indicate the curvature of the whole spine. The reader can make up one's own key. The important thing is to be able to capture and notate the structural alignment that one is seeing as quickly as possible.

The example ideogram (Fig. 93) shows a low right buttock, high left hip, buttock crease points slightly to the left, the lumbar spine is shifted to the left with an opposing shift to the right in the thoracic spine, a skin fold on the left side at the diaphragm level, a low left shoulder and a head tilted to the left. The arrow on the left side above the pelvis indicates a left side anterior pelvic rotation, the dotted line indicates the plumb line position consistent with the rotation of the pelvis but the plumb is central further up. The plus signs indicate tight bulging muscles in left scapula and left buttock area and the negative signs indicate a weakness in the right buttock muscles

One thing to remember, when doing structural body reading from the back, is that it is the *first impression* that counts. The longer you look the more inclined you are to alter your opinion on what you think you are seeing. This often happens because, without being aware of it, one unconsciously moves the position of one's head or body and one loses one's line of sight. Also, the longer the client is standing on the board the more likely the client is to move about.

Dr. Stone points out a few common distortions of the body in his books and how the body tends to adapt as he learned from his typical clients. But the reader should also remember that he said that any distortion or abnormality is possible in a client.

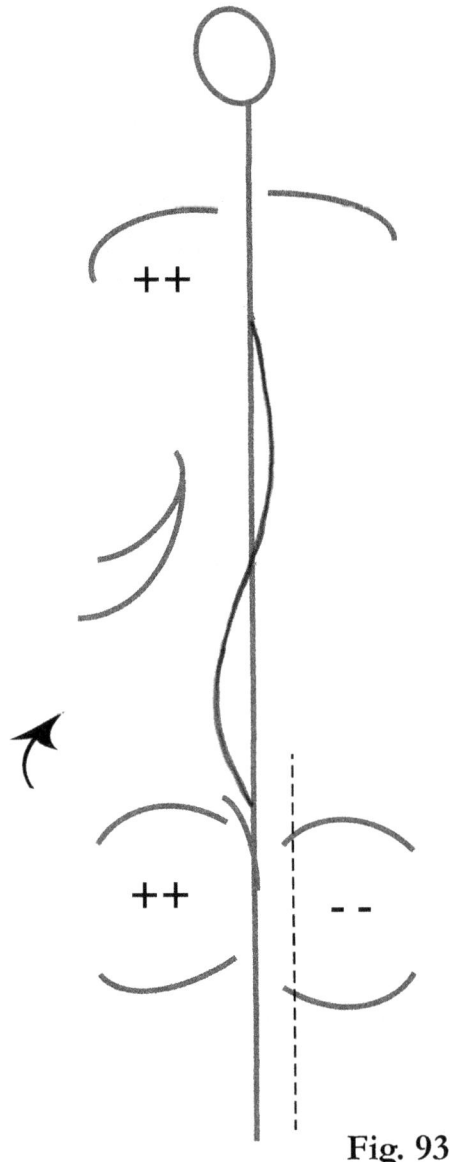

Fig. 93

In relation to the plumb line, he also wrote:

> The findings and varieties are many and too involved to picture all of them. The factors behind all this are not only the muscles under tension, but the impulses to these muscles from fields of sensory abdominal reflexes and emotional stress.
>
> Vol. I, Book 3, p. 66

It is this that makes it really difficult to generalize when talking about structural work. For example, he says that an anterior-inferior sacral base on either side usually creates the short leg and low shoulder on the same side. He also says that the anterior-inferior sacral base side is also the side of the body that moves anterior unless (and here is the essence of the problem) there are other complicating twists and distortions or where, over a period of time, the natural compensatory function of the body has changed this situation.

Fig. 94 shows the typical result of a tilt of the sacral base as described above. The sacral base is tilted to the right, creating a low right shoulder and a general contraction on that side of the body. The sacral position is indicated by the right buttock being lower than the left. The actual sacral position shown is greatly exaggerated for clarity. In this situation, the right side of the body is often anterior (left side posterior), as indicated by the fact that the plumb line is falling to the left of the centre line. In this example, the minus signs indicate the anterior side of the body, and the plus signs the posterior side (not muscle tension). In clients who have excess body fat at waist level there is often a crease on the opposite side of the body to that in which the sacrum is tilting; in this case the skin crease or fold is on the left side. Though the skin fold can be on the same side as the low sacral base, the position of the fold largely depends on what the lumbar spine is doing. Is the lumbar spine

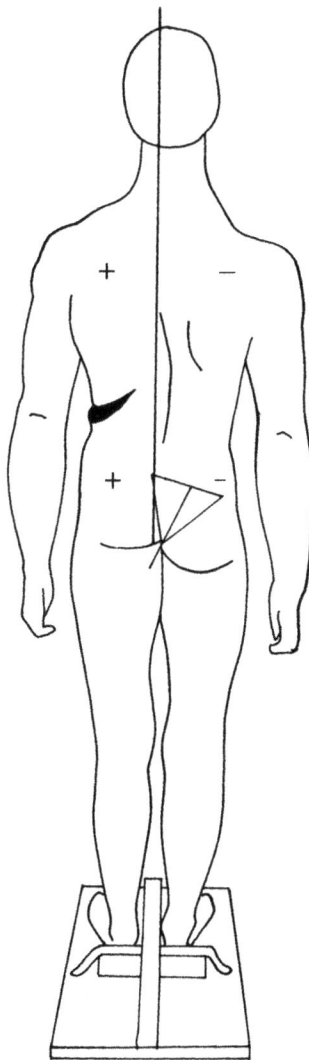

Fig. 94

accommodating the movement of the sacrum by moving to the same side as the low sacral base (as in this example making a concave curvature to the right) or has it moved to the opposite side (making a curvature to the left)?

> The plumb line shows distortions and muscle tensions that are unequal in the skeletal framework. A patient can be badly distorted and yet not be very sick; he may not even know it. Another patient may check good on the plumb line, and can feel terribly bad.
>
> The plumb line does not indicate vital function distortions, nor Sympathetic or Parasympathetic nerve disturbances, nor acute inflammatory diseases, except when skeletal muscles are involved. The plumb line is a good check for <u>structural</u> distortions, but <u>not for functional imbalance</u>. There are many lines of stress in the body energy fields that are not governed by mere physical gravity. The four elements themselves are beyond the law of gravity, as they are energy particles of the finest kind, a fourth grade of matter, like electrons.
>
> Vol. II, Book 5, p. 59

So, it is important to remember that the gravity board is no kind of indicator of the client's overall state of health. If a client is complaining of severe lower back pains and yet lines up straight and level on the gravity board, then, as Dr. Stone points out in his writings, one may probably be dealing with prostatic trouble if it is a male client or uterine disturbance in a female. The key factor to remember is that the life energy is beyond the influence of gravity, and so the body's relationship to gravity is not a useful guide to the health of the client. Please bear in mind that *structurally corrective techniques are not given when there is acute pain and inflammation.* It is vital to reduce the inflammation and pain first, through releasing the related energy blocks, before trying to make structural corrections.

A structural bodywork session can be a little unusual in its organisation in that part way through the session the practitioner may ask the client to stand up so that their body can be read again using the gravity board. This allows the practitioner to evaluate the effectiveness of the corrective impulses being given to the client's body and to change them if necessary.

As I mentioned earlier, it is really helpful to practice structure reading first on all one's clients before doing standard elemental, reflex or nervous system work. Doing this takes away the stress of thinking one needs to get it right because one is about to do a session based on one's reading. Practicing this procedure allows one time to develop body-reading skills. Body reading is an art in itself and one worth pursuing. One thing that I found most helpful was to train my eyes on an everyday basis. I did this by reading peoples bodies in the street as I walked behind them. I also did it whilst sitting in cafés. I would read people as they walked in and out of the main door, as the door frame gave good vertical and horizontal reference markers by which to evaluate their structure. All this helps to increase the accuracy of one's mental snapshots of the structure.

One thing that is a challenge for some students learning structural work, is the emotional issue of feeling that one has to do something right, to evaluate the structure correctly and do appropriate work to get structural change. The challenge is how one deals with failure. In the general practice of Polarity Therapy, the practitioner gives the client a session and does not really know the outcome of that session until the client comes back a week later for their next appointment. In some cases, of course, there may only be a small change, but this does not mean the practitioner has failed or that there has to be a sense of failure in relation to the previous session. Most Polarity Therapists just view a session that did not have much positive impact on the client as simply part of a larger process where there are peaks and troughs as the energy reacts to the work being done. There is perhaps the awareness of the need to do something different, but there is not any sense of having failed.

What has just been said applies to the energetic component. The same thing is not true of the structural work because one re-evaluates changes that have taken place in the structure both during and immediately after the session. Sometimes the structure simply does not respond to one's work. When that happens one is staring failure in the face. I suspect it is why some Polarity practitioners never delve into the structural work because it can be a very uncomfortable practice. Recall what we discussed in Chapter 1 about the practitioner's attitude to the work. This is the type of work where the use of the neutral attitude as espoused by Pierre Pannetier is the most appropriate one to adopt.

Perhaps the most fundamental reason that structural work might not create change is when the client is deeply invested in their identity as it is. The second most common cause may be that, in spite of the pain and discomfort caused by the structural pattern, it may be affording a kind of secondary gain whereby the psychological or practical benefits of the distortional pattern outweigh the value of changing it. A simple example could be when a painful back gives a person the practical benefit of being able to take time off from work, particularly if the client finds work less than rewarding except financially.

Treatment Strategies

Preparatory Technique:

Before using any structural techniques, it is vital that one always release the front of the body first. When I first heard this concept, it sounded like a rule and, since I was of a mildly anarchic mindset, I felt I had to challenge the rule by doing some sessions where I went straight into structural technique on the back of the body. I vividly remember one experience when I worked on a male client who had a serious degree of pelvic imbalance with accompanying distortion in the spine, shoulder girdle and head/neck balance. I put him face down on the table after the body reading and got to work. After about thirty minutes I had him stand up and re-checked his structure using the gravity board and everything looked wonderfully resolved. The pelvis and shoulders had become level, the spine straightened and the head was in much better balance. As I had 10 minutes left, I got him back on the table on his back so I could do some very gentle work on the front of the body. At the end of the session I checked him again and everything had gone back to the original imbalance! To say I was shocked is to put it mildly. After a couple of other similar experiences, I decided that to *release the front of the body first* really was a useful rule in structural bodywork. It took me some time to realise why this is the case. The answer lies in the sensory/motor feedback from the front to the back of the body.

In Polarity theory, the front of the body is sensory and the back is motor. In any sensory/motor feedback system the sensory always dominates the motor aspect. Think of a thermostat that controls a boiler: the thermostat (the sensory system) controls the boiler (the motor system). It does this through a simple thermocouple that feeds an electrical impulse to an on/off switch that controls the boiler. Any structural distortion on the back of the body is held in place and controlled by the sensory impulses coming from the front.

If you just release the back of the body, the lightest interaction with the front will immediately send those old patterned sensory impulses to the back of the body again. This will instantly force the pattern on the back of the body to resume its original relationship with the front. By releasing the front of the body first you are, in essence, doing a system reset which will allow your work on the back of the body to find a new improved relationship with the activity on the front of the body after the session is over. By releasing the front of the body first you are breaking the sensory/motor feedback loop that maintains the imbalance. Oddly, on my many detailed readings of Dr. Stone's work I did not find this rule stated anywhere—yet it is a profoundly valuable understanding.

> Structure reacts from the bottom, up and is therefore a major for any structural correction or balance.
>
> Vol. II, Book 5, p. 19

> If it is the Life Currents which we are trying to influence, then the superior pole is the most influential. But, if it is structure the inferior pole or foundation will be more in line with the proposition and with the principle of gravity pull.

> Life flows from above downward, and structure supports function from below upward. Life is the first impulse. Reaction is the second wave, which must return to make a circle or a circuit of energy flow as CAUSE AND EFFECT, or positive and negative poles of the current.
>
> Vol. II, Book 4, p. 3

> Impulse from above supplies the structure. And structure imbalance from below perverts natural impulse by blocking its flow.
>
> Vol. II, 25 Charts. Chart 20

In the above quotes, where Dr. Stone talks about working from the bottom up, he is advocating the same release of the sensory pole prior to working on the motor pole. This being in relation to the primary polarity of top/bottom where the top is the positive motor pole and the bottom is sensory negative pole. A simple way of speaking of the importance of the work on the lower body lies in that simple statement that we mentioned earlier: *a house rests on, and is only as good as, its foundation.*

Key points in Structural Treatment:

1. Read the structural alignment of the body using the gravity board and plumb line. If you do not have access to these, you can still do some structural reading of the body by visually checking the alignment of the heels and checking to see which is the short-leg side and beginning the work based on those indicators. It is also possible to check many of the primary sacral indicators such as hip and shoulder position without a gravity board. You can also use motion testing.

2. Release the front of the body first. You can use relaxed hand contacts working with or against the long-line current flow as well as 5-pointed star technique to release the psoas/iliacus complex.

3. Work from the bottom up, i.e. begin at the feet and finish at the head.

4. Establish a functional balance in the feet before working up through the structure.

5. Use the tri-axial geometry—top/bottom, left/right and front/back balancing. Most of the work you do will probably focus on the first two sets of these three primary polarities.

6. A simple free-form structural session is to cross relate and re-polarise tension areas as seen on the gravity board.

7. Make sure you are fully conversant with perineal and coccyx work so that you can address the autonomic nervous systems impact on the structure. Dr. Stone would often precede any structural work with a perineal session.

8. Use directional contacts, study Figures 74-76.

9. When working on the spine and specific vertebrae, release the related negative poles in the feet first (see p. 232).

10. When doing any work on the head and neck by such techniques as the North Pole Stretch, please be aware of the following comment from Dr. Stone:

> Techniques of reflex therapy which release causes of the energy blocks from below *should be used first before any attempt* is made to treat or to adjust the neck. [Italics added.]
>
> Vol. I, Book 2, Chart 41

During the Session:

By now it is evident that a unique feature of a structural session is that one will probably re-read the body structure either by getting the client off the table to stand on the gravity board or by re-evaluating through other assessment procedures such as motion testing and checking the heels and short-leg side. These assessment procedures enable one to evaluate whether the treatment strategy is effective or not. If the treatment is not producing the change one is looking for, as evidenced by these structural evaluations, one has the opportunity to work in a different way for the remainder of the session. In my own work, I will typically re-read the body using motion tests many times throughout a session.

After the Session:

One of the most important issues at the end of a structural session is persuading the client not to test his or her structure. It is common for a client with a bad back to get off the table after treatment and start testing his or her back by twisting and stretching this way and that to discover if there is less pain. *It is vital that the client be prevented from doing this.* Stopping the client will require explaining in detail why it is necessary to slowly get off the table without contortions, step onto the gravity board so their body structure can be re-read, and thereafter to sit quietly for a few minutes.

Explain all this to the client before beginning the bodywork. Then remind the client again at the end of the bodywork before the client gets up off the table. Experience has shown me that a client needs to be in a somewhat neutral relationship with gravity for at least five minutes after they get off the table. This allows for the central nervous system and energy to integrate and stabilise the new alignment relative to the pull of gravity. Challenging it sooner will tend to break up the new patterning. By the time one has re-read the client's body and had the person sit and discuss follow-up sessions, possible treatment reactions and so forth, this period for re-integration will pass quickly. Make sure the client does not try to put shoes and socks on while one is talking, until the full five minutes have passed.

After re-reading the client's body structure at the end of the session, it is almost inevitable that a client will ask "how it looks." What the client means is whether there is any improvement. No matter what one sees, one should always say it has improved. There is no point in telling the client that his or her structure is unchanged, even if one is seeing no improvement. While saying there is improvement when one cannot see any might seem disingenuous, it is vital that the client maintain a positive attitude towards the sessions.

There are some curiosities in what can be seen when re-reading the client's body after a session. Often I have experienced immense shock at the level of change I have seen when looking at the body at the end of the session, only to realise when I re-checked all the specific parameters that I had notated at the beginning that they were, in fact, unchanged! Nothing actually changed structurally due to the treatment. My understanding of this process is that, as my mind compares the new "snapshot" of the client's physical structure with the initial one, I am picking up a global shift in either the client's energy, emotionality or identity being expressed through his or her structure, even though the structure has not as yet changed physically. Saying it another way: even though the relationship of the structural parts is the same, the gestalt of the whole has transformed in some dramatic way.

Another thing often seen is that the pelvis, which may have been higher on one side before treatment, has now shifted into exactly the opposite orientation, now being high on the other side of the body rather than having moved into level balance. In my early practice, I tended to think of this as being the effect of the release of a tension pattern going into an oscillation, as a stretched rubber band that is released will oscillate back and forth until it finally stabilises in a neutral position. Now I understand this kind of change in the pelvis as being related to a re-building of energy from depletion into a more active state as the person realigns with his or her gender identity which is an important part of our total identity.

It is quite common for clients who have had physical therapy to ask if there are any exercises they can or should do and I always recommend against this, telling them that exercise is best left until after they are more balanced structurally and pain-free. Exercise can often be yet another negative physical stress that can cause further problematic structural compensations. It can add new layers or strengthen existing compensations, depending on the type of exercise.

Some General Considerations:

Early in my practice I had a male client in his fifties who was a farmer. He worked a small holding, digging the fields by hand. This in itself is not remarkable were it not for the fact that he was born with achondroplasic dwarfism. He had all the typical characteristics of this condition: short arms and legs, large head and extreme lumbar lordosis.

Understandably, he came for treatment of back pain. After few months of structural treatment combined with dietary reform, his chronic back pain resolved nicely. Near the end of the time I worked him, at the beginning of one of our sessions, he remarked that my treatments were expensive. I was somewhat surprised at the comment and said so to him. His response was that it was not that my treatments were too expensive. Rather, as he put it, "You know how everyone has a pair of shoes that they have had for years. It's like they are old friends. Well, I put my old shoes on the other day and my back immediately became painful, so I took them off. I looked at the soles and noticed that they were really worn down on one side. So, I threw them out and bought some new shoes. That is why I said your session were expensive, as I have had to buy new shoes!" All this he conveyed to me with a chuckle. It was a powerful learning experience for me and I began looking carefully at the shoes of all my structural clients. I realised that a worn shoe is, in itself, a kind of passive machine that can work exactly like an orthotic lift. The wear pattern reflects and can re-instate a structural pattern that you are trying to resolve. So now, if I see a lot of wear, I always recommend the client get some new shoes which have neutral structural patterning. Some modern shoes have very strong soles that resist wear, but check the inside because one will often see that the foot bed has collapsed or become distorted. In that case, the insole must be replaced.

It is common for clients with long-standing structural issues and pain to have been prescribed orthotic lifts. It is a thorny question as to what to say about orthotics. My preference is the client not use orthotics for at least two or three structural sessions. Ultimately, I leave the choice up to them, merely expressing my preference. Most clients seem happy not to use them.

Dr Stone's Approach

In his books, Dr. Stone does not give any examples of a full structural session beginning with a body reading and then on through a treatment process. However, the session he outlined below is instructive. It is a sacroiliac balance sequence from Vol. II, Book 5, p. 68. The bracketed sections in italics contain my commentary on the session:

The treatment employed:

1. The perineal contact, together with its POLARITY balance contact in the neck, the shoulders and the sorest spot in the back, until complete relaxation has occurred and the

pulse is balanced. This indicates the re-establishment of the flow of 'Prana' to the blocked energy fields, and the short leg will be lengthened.

(Dr. Stone's tended to follow a standard sequence for perineal work. He always began with the related neck contacts to the disturbed side of the perineum. Then the contacts on the shoulders address the 11th cranial nerve—the spinal accessory nerve with its resonances to the parasympathetic nervous system—and then finally to the sorest area on the back. Dr. Stone often just treated the most tender area on the perineum and the back as the location of the most potent energetic locks which, when released, normally clear the larger local area. More areas than just the sorest one can be treated if one desires, but this is a treatment strategy based upon the most economical usage of time within the format of the relatively short session duration that Dr. Stone, as an osteopath, used. This would typically have been between 20 and 30 minutes when he was in private practice.)

2. The gluteal soreness and spasms are balanced with the shoulders and the spinal soreness and spasms.

(See Fig. 75 and Fig. 76 on p. 169 and the instructions at "A" and "B" on using the thumbs as directional contacts.)

3. The psoas magnus, the iliacus, and the rectus abdominalis will now be found less sore than before, and partly relaxed. Inhibition will complete the relaxing process in a few minutes.

(The practitioner can check for this release by having the client turn over and testing around Poupart's ligament (The modern term for the Poupart's ligament is the inguinal ligament) or by gently lifting one's fingertips into this same area if the client is face down. However, to inhibit and fully relax this area, the practitioner needs to turn the client over on to their back. See Fig. 74, p. 168 and the description on p. 167 for Dr. Stone's approach in detail.)

4.Balance the functional leverage strain in front of the body, from the acetabulum on one side to the shoulder on the other side.

(The client is now on his or her back. This manipulation should be familiar as a type of 5-pointed star treatment that works farther out near the outside edge of the body in the region around the hip joint rather than from Poupart's ligament and the soft tissue immediately above the ligament.)

5. Structural correction of the 5th lumbar [L5], the sacrum, the ilium, etc. can now be made and maintained naturally by the sympathetic nervous system.

(Dr. Stone indicates that, even though his background is osteopathic, no force is necessary to correct the relationship between sacrum and L5. The rebalancing of the autonomic nervous system will cause muscular relaxation in the pelvis which will, in turn, facilitate the natural repositioning of these structures via normal everyday movement. Indeed, it would be quite normal for you to hear a soft click from the lower back, indicating a release in some of the facet joints of the spine, as the client gets off the table or when bending forward to put on their shoes.)

In the following section, the specific structural manipulations are based upon a body-reading of an actual client, so that the directional aspect of the techniques can be clearly related to the body-reading.

For me, the structural balancing aspect of Polarity Therapy is more art form than science. Some Polarity Therapists love this type of work, with all its inherent challenges and contradictions, while others are happier working with the "wireless anatomy," the elemental, reflex or neurological approaches to Polarity bodywork. My personal passion is structural work. Whatever approach the reader uses, if one goes deeply enough, one will evolve an artful form of bodywork.

9. STRUCTURAL BALANCING TECHNIQUES

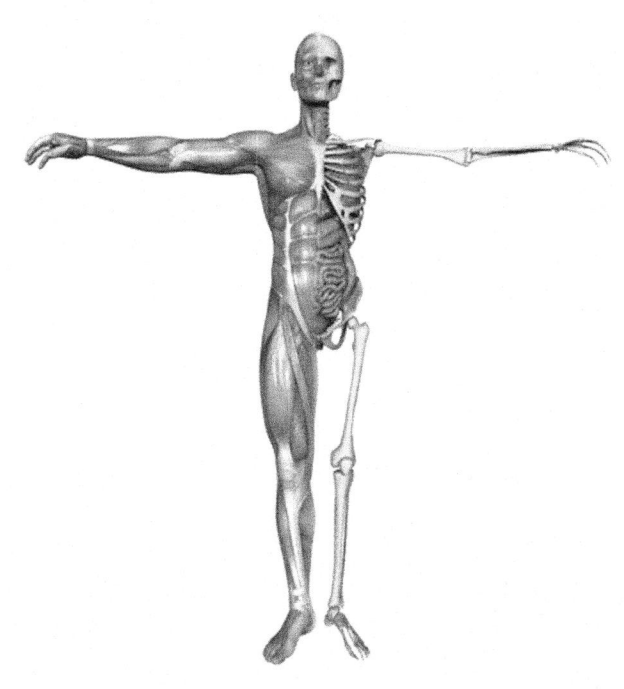

Client - Body Reading

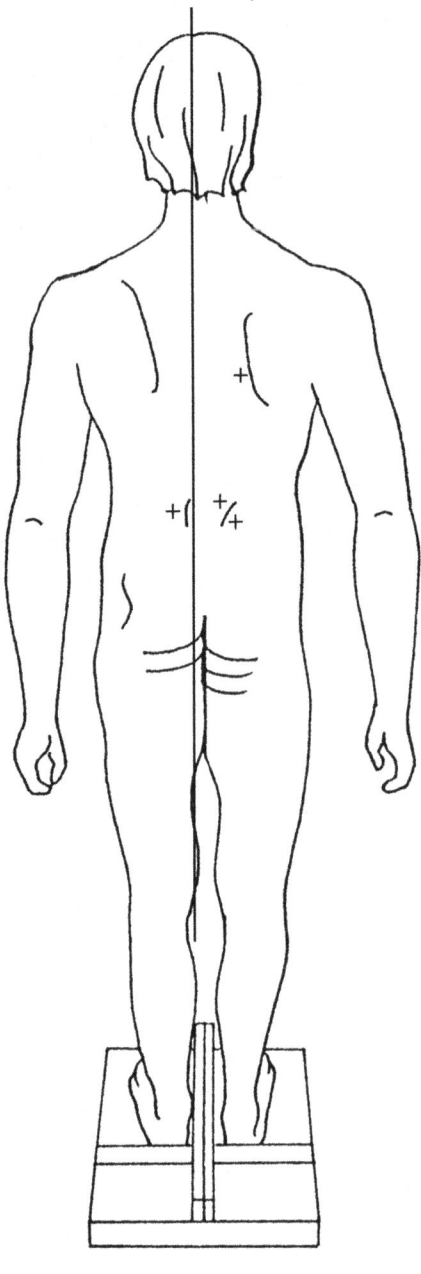

Fig. 95

Fig. 95 is a drawing of the structural alignment of an actual client on the gravity board. This same client is the model used for the structural balancing treatments that follow. Whilst it is not written up as an illustrated case history study, I will make some comments throughout on the kind of changes that took place, as well as a more detailed look at the end on the overall changes after three sessions of structural bodywork. Looking at the figure, the first thing to note from the buttock level line is that the sacral base is inferior and anterior on the right side. The body is rotated anterior on the right, as shown by the plumb line falling to the left of the centre line. The left iliac crest is a little high. Note the tension in the left gluteal muscles. The right shoulder is dropped, which is most noticeable from the crease at the armpit rather than the top line of the shoulders and the difference in the position of the scapula. Note the different way the arms hang on each side of the body and the breadth of the upper body relative to the pelvis. There is also a lot of muscular tension near the right scapula and in the lumbar area on both sides (marked with plus signs). Lastly the plumb line indicates no spinal compensation for the sacral position and the head is also in line with the spine. This last fact is most interesting because it means that his body has at least a tertiary layer of compensation overlaid on top of the secondary compensation that occurs when the sacrum is out of position. The client had injured himself some months previously carrying a heavy weight, and was experiencing quite a lot of pain in the sacrum when both stationary and in movement.

The Foundation - Feet

A structural session always begins at the feet, as a structure is truly only as good as its foundation. There are two arches in the foot, the longitudinal and the transverse. The longitudinal arch is shown on the left of Fig. 96 and the transverse in the middle. On the right it shows how the transverse arch of each foot forms a complete structure when taken together. Fallen arches in the foot can have a profound effect upon the structure of the body, however in most cases the reason for the fallen arch is not due to bone misalignment but to muscular weakness in the foot and lower legs, which often needs to be addressed by exercise to strengthen the weak muscles. It is important that any energy blocks in the feet should be resolved before you do anything else. Dr. Stone talked of creating a functional balance in the feet before doing any structural work.

Correction for a Low Arch

This technique and the following one are osteopathic manipulation of the bones of the feet designed to reposition the specific bones that form the arches and that are out of place due to some kind of injury, such as can be caused by everything from a simple misstep off a pavement or step to more serious trauma such as having your foot trodden

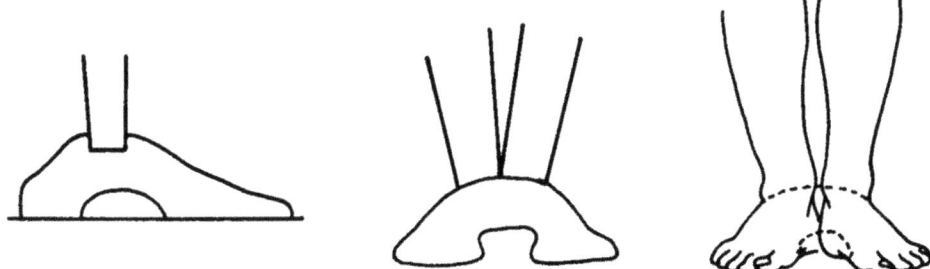

Fig. 96

on or run over. It is vital that you do not treat these just as physical technique but as always with Polarity Therapy and in keeping with Dr. Stone's phrase, "old moves with a new impetus" the energetic dimension needs to be addressed by holding the foot and sensing the energy between your hands before trying the particular manipulation.

Manipulating the bones of the feet can have a powerful effect upon the whole of the body because the feet are the major negative pole of the body and have reflexes to all the major organs and correcting the arches can help to relieve pain and muscular discomfort due to structural imbalance.

Client is on their back

1. Stand at the client's feet.
2. To treat the right foot, grip the arch of the foot firmly with your right hand (Fig. 97), and with your left hand grip the outside of the foot so that the fingers support the heel and the palm covers the cuboid bone with the thumb below the ankle bone (Fig. 98).

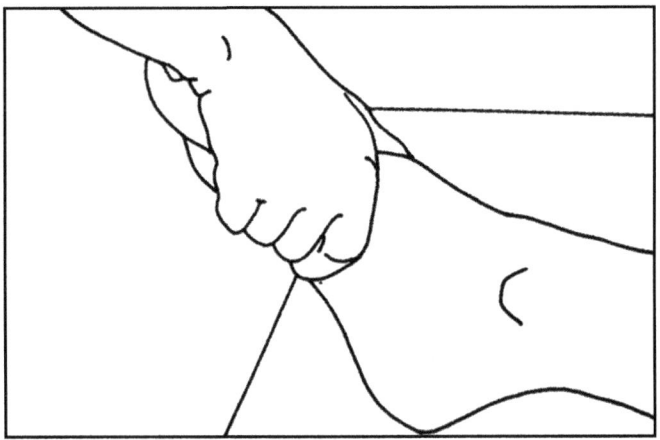

Fig. 97

3. Hold each contact firmly until you can feel the energy flowing strongly and then the arch correction is a simultaneous twist of the right hand and a quick short thrust of the left hand to the right. See directional arrows in Fig. 98.

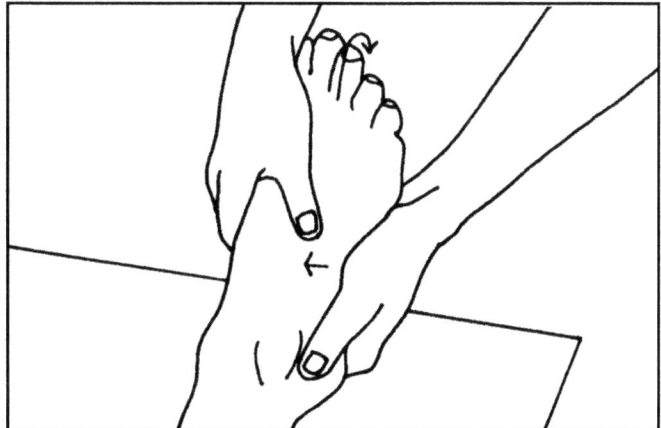

Fig. 98

Correction for a High Arch

This is a specific adjustment for a high arch in the foot but it is a beneficial technique for the whole leg as it causes a gentle separation of the joints of the ankle, knee and hip. The hand position on top of the foot reflexes to the middle back. The technique can be done slightly lower on the foot (closer to the ankle) with the middle finger influencing the cuboid bone, in which case it is a powerful stimulation of the kidney area. It can also be used to re-position the talus and the tibia bones if there is difficulty in ankle flexion due to bone misalignment. When pulling the leg, only use enough force to effectively separate and free the joints, relying on the body's self regulating ability to affect re-alignment where necessary.

Client is on their back

1. Stand at client's feet.
2. Grasp the right foot with both your hands. Your palms are overlapped on the instep of the foot. Your thumbs are below the ball of the foot (Fig. 99 overleaf).
3. Ask client to inhale. As they do, flex their foot as you bend it towards their head.
4. Ask them to exhale. Just before they have exhaled all the air in their lungs, and with the foot still flexed, pull the entire leg towards you 3/4 inch or 2 cm. It is a quick short pull in the direction of the arrow in Fig. 99. Hold this position for several seconds and then release your grip.

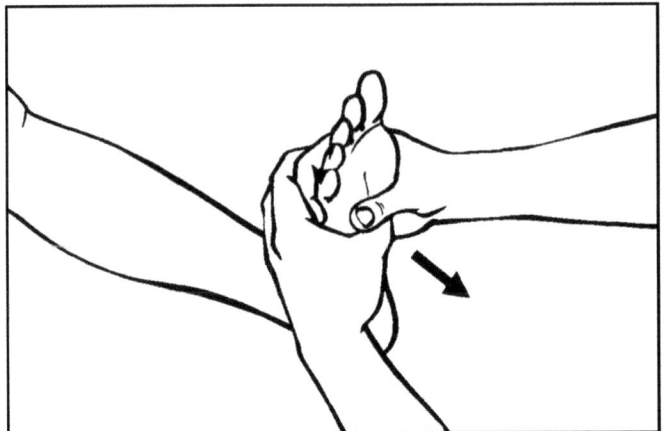

Fig. 99

Os Calcis Correction

The os calcis bone or calcaneum is the foundation bone of the body structure. It is the negative pole of the occiput, the sacrum being the neuter pole. There is very often tenderness around the heel on the short leg side and severe occipital tension on the opposite side, though occasionally the occipital tension manifests on the same side. It is usually the heel bone on the short leg side that is most distorted, and so the technique is usually done on the short leg side. However, both ankles can be out of line in which case both are treated. Fig. 100 shows as a straight line the pull of gravity from the heel bones through the sacro-iliac articulation to the occiput, and as dotted lines the energy waves radiating from the occiput down through the muscles of the back through the hip joints to the heels. The integrity of these lines of energy determines, in part, the posture in relation to gravity. The left side of Fig. 100 shows the relationship between the force of gravity and the energy waves as being like the rigging of a ship's mast, which is the only way to stabilize a tall structure like the body. As we explored earlier the os calcis correction has all the necessary elements of *a general session for the structure*. Specifically, it has a great deal of effect on body rotation, the body frequently rotates anterior on the inferior anterior sacral base side. The rotational aspect is significant in that the rotation seen in most structural distortion involves a screwing down, in the same way that a top can be screwed down on a jar. The structure loses elasticity as the rotation tends to shorten and tighten the body. Pragmatically speaking, I cannot stress the importance of this session enough, in relation to structural correction because, as I explained in the last chapter, it constitutes a general session for the structure.

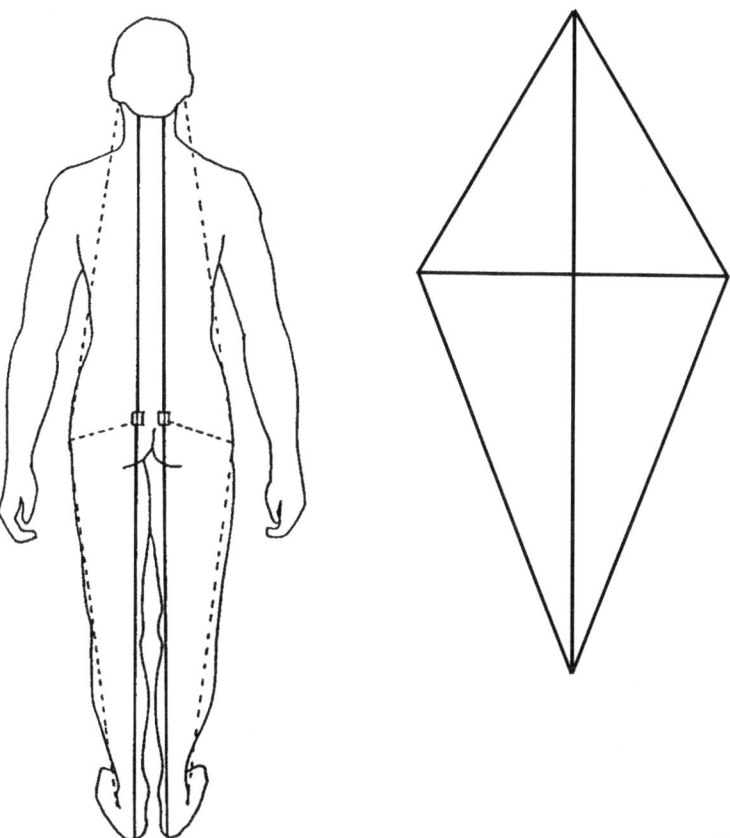

Fig. 100

211

Normal heel positioning allows free movement of the ankle in either direction (Fig. 101). A typical distortion is seen in Fig. 102 and this is also the actual position of the os calcis bones of our client. It is the heel of the client's short leg side that is the most distorted.

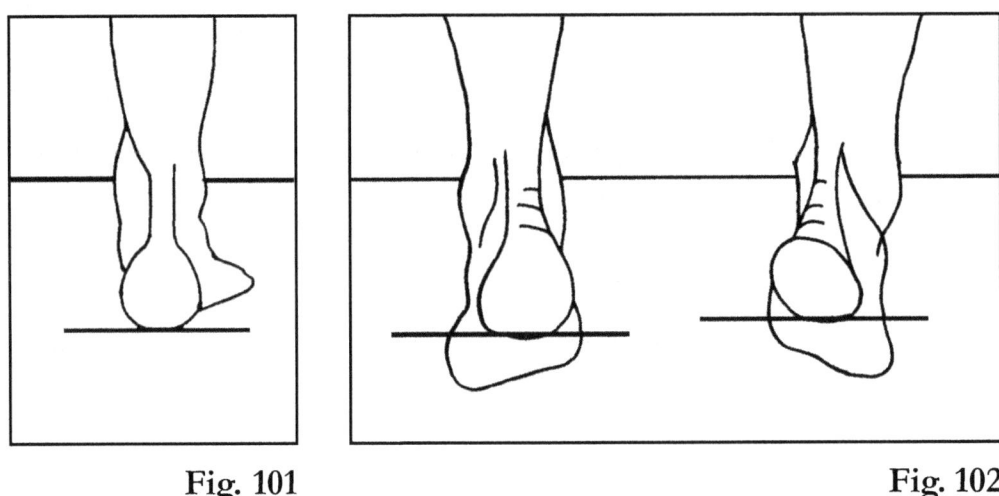

Fig. 101   **Fig. 102**

Client is on their front

1. Stand on his right side.
2. Raise the right foot, and with your right thumb contact the sorest point just above the heel on the outside of the os calcis bone. The fingers are placed over the heel base so that the tips rest on the inside of the heel.
3. Contact the diaphragm reflex area on the foot with the thumb of your left hand (Fig. 103).

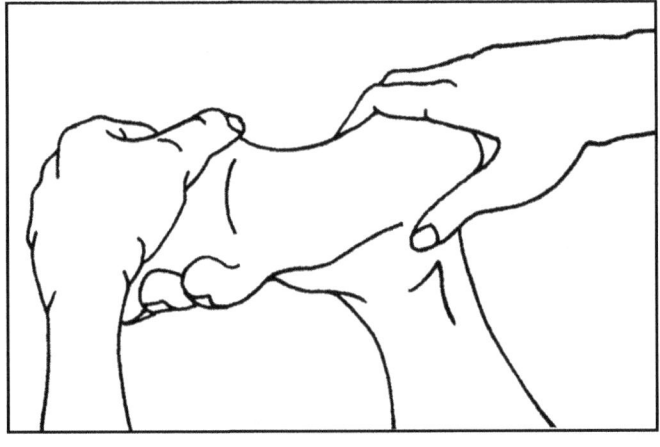

Fig. 103

4. Alternately stimulate the diaphragm reflex with a circular movement while holding the heel bone in an outwards direction, maintaining the thumb pressure on the sore spot. Do this for 1-2 minutes until you can feel the energy strongly.
5. Lay the leg down and make the same corrective heel contact but this time with the left hand, and with the right hand explore the calf, working on any tight muscles you feel there using either your thumb or fingertips using either gentle rajasic work or inhibiting the tense muscles. Then rock the client's right thigh in the same direction (in particular any tense muscle groups). Stimulate the calf and the thigh for 1-2 minutes on each until you can feel the energy flowing.
6. Keeping the same heel contact, move the right hand up to the hip joint and contact any tight muscles around the joint with your fingertips. Stimulate for 1-2 minutes until you feel the muscles release and the energy flowing strongly (Fig. 104).

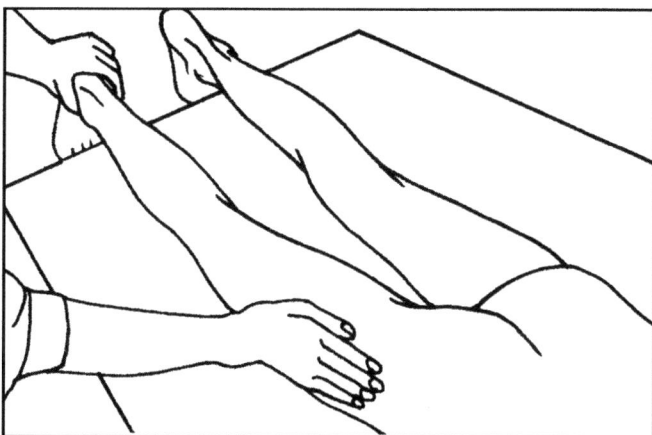

Fig. 104

7. Still holding the heel, move your right hand to the client's right sacro-iliac articulation. Stimulate the sacral joint for 1-2 minutes (Fig. 105).

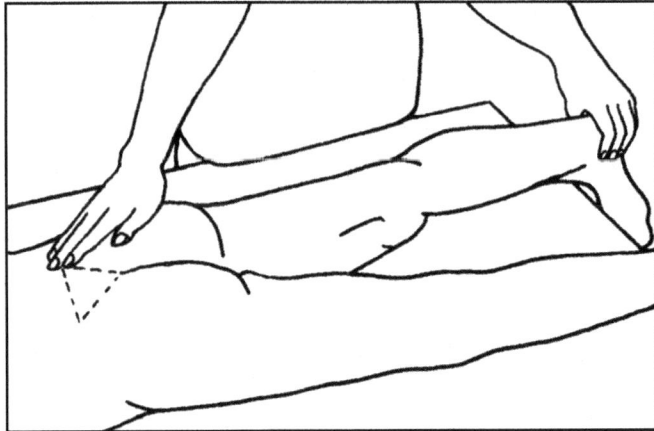

Fig. 105

8. Move the right hand up the body to contact any tense areas on the back (marked with a plus sign). Stimulate them as you hold the heel for 1-2 minutes. To do this effectively you may need to bend the leg at the knee.

9. Contact the sorest side of the occipital ridge. In this case it is the client's left side. Stimulate the occiput as you hold the heel contact for 1-2 minutes until the tenderness eases (Fig. 106).

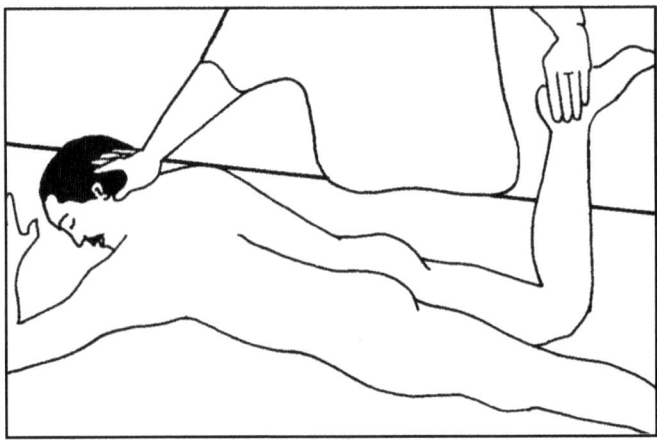

Fig. 106

If the client's heel is twisting outwards the sore spot to work will be located on the inside of the heel. The correction, no matter what the distortion, is always to level the heel base and realign it.

At this point place the client's feet back on the bolster or just over the edge of the couch and you should find the heels are level. If you want to you can ask them to stand on the gravity board again so that you can see how this session has changed the overall structure. In keeping with our concept of the os calcis correction being a general treatment for the structure I have had clients whose whole structure has realigned after one such treatment. In this particular case, the rotation in the client's structure vanished but little else changed.

Short Leg Correction

The short leg is indicative of an overall contraction in the energy currents on that side of the body. When any of the six primary polarities in the body (top/bottom, left/right, front/back) are out of balance it is a major impediment to the self-healing and self-balancing capacities of the body. Dr. Stone said that when the short leg side lengthens and stays long it indicates that normal repair processes are able to take place within the body. It would also indicate that the sacrum was level and that the muscular and energetic forces around it are balanced, as the short leg side is caused by sacral distortion and muscular imbalance in the pelvis. To be precise, Dr. Stone indicated that a shift in the sacral position is the primary cause of the short leg. For example, a right anterior inferior sacral base, as the primary factor, will immediately cause a compensation of the pelvis whereby the innominate moves up on that right side in an attempt to bring the sacrum level so that it is not load bearing. It is this compensatory shift in the innominate position that gives the short leg reading. To make things even more complicated, it is quite possible for further shifts in the sacrum to occur, necessitating more compensatory shifts in the innominate position. Thus, you can have an initial right short leg followed by another later set of compensations that cause the appearance of a left short leg. In that scenario you have, in essence, two short leg patterns.

There are various techniques[1] that release the short leg side and they can be done independently of a full structural balancing session. For instance, the following short leg technique can be incorporated into a normal general energy balancing session if required.

A short leg correction, as a specific technique, need not be done during a session that has a structural orientation, as any work to re-balance the sacral position will always correct the short leg.

Short Leg Release by Torque

The short leg side is often the tense leg side. To determine the short and tense leg have the client on their back and with your air fingers simultaneously push each foot towards the centre line of the body (medial rotation) and compare the tension, and resistance to

---

1. See *Polarity Therapy-Healing with Life Energy* by Alan Siegel M.S. N.D. and Phil Young, p. 141 for other techniques.

movement. The leg that is most difficult to move is the short and tense leg. Returning to our client whose short and tense leg is the right:

Client is on their back

1. Stand on the client's right side.
2. Pick up and rotate the right leg medially (towards the centre line) and hold in this position by having the left hand on the thigh and the right hand below the knee (Fig. 107).

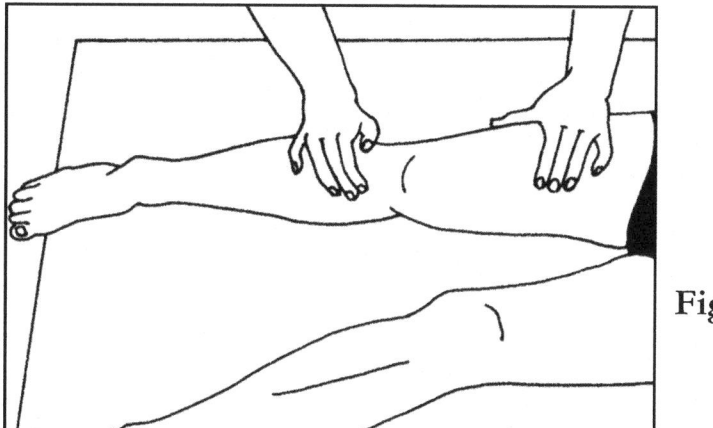

Fig. 107

3. Holding the leg in this position, rock it gently and rhythmically towards the centre line. The whole body should begin to rock gently. Continue rocking for 2-3 minutes until the muscles release.

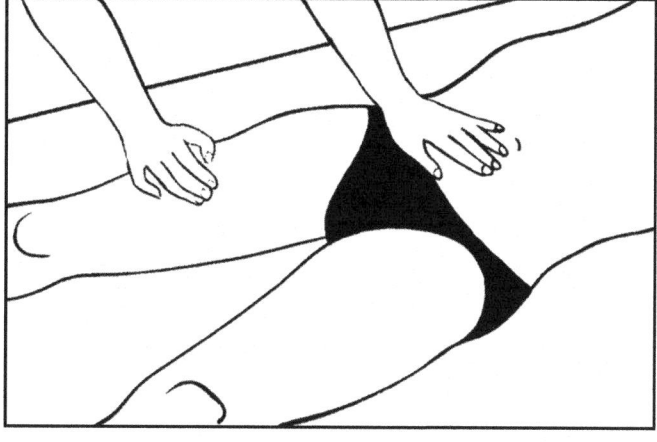

Fig. 108

4. The hand positions can be changed during the treatment, moving up and down the leg but still keeping it medially rotated. It is particularly beneficial to release the thigh muscles in relation to the anterior pelvic muscles, still rocking the leg inwards (Fig. 108, previous page).

In this short leg technique we used a motion test to establish the short leg side. However, the most common way to check leg length is to compare various bones in the feet (Fig. 109). You can compare many of the bones in the feet, left to right and also the position of the heels with the feet flexed. I find the most accurate indicator is the internal or medial malleolus. Before checking for leg length difference it is helpful to move each leg out to the side by about 18 inches or 45 cm and give the leg a gentle pull. This will release any fixation between the head of the femur and the acetabulum that might interfere with an accurate short leg reading. Short leg readings can be taken with the client face up or face down.

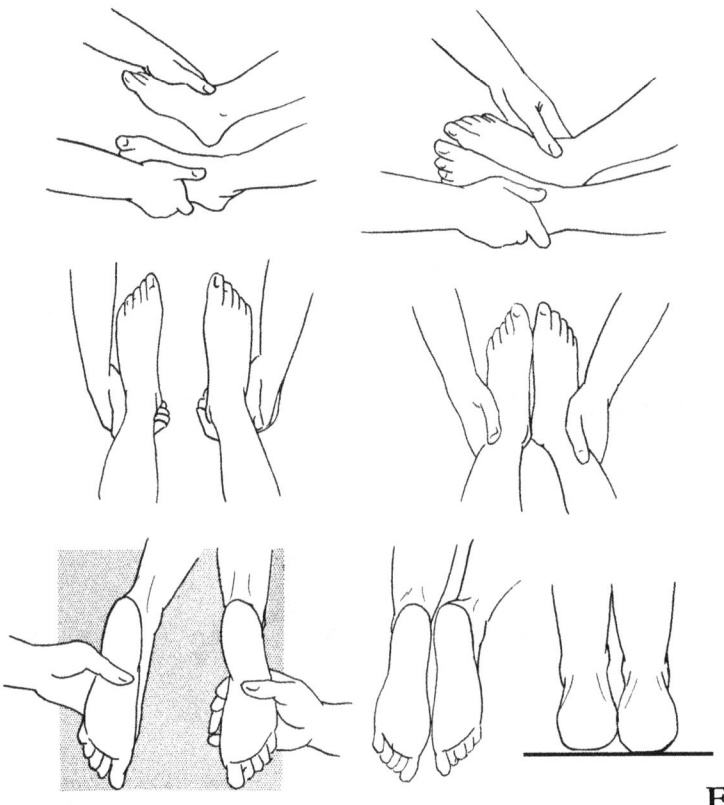

Fig. 109

Sacral Corrections

The sacrum is the focal point where all the physical stresses and strains and the force of gravity meet in the body. We have already explored in detail the role of the sacrum as a keystone structure in the body and its role in the whole structural balancing process. Architecturally speaking, apart from the sacrum being a keystone in the arch of the pelvis, the whole pelvic area also acts as a cantilever type structure. A common example of a cantilever is a diving spring board, anchored at one end supporting the weight of the diver at the other. A cantilever bridge is another example, in these structures the cantilevers are commonly built in pairs, with each cantilever used to support one end of a central section.

Fig. 110 shows the architectural structure of the relationship between the sacrum and the hip joints as a cantilever.

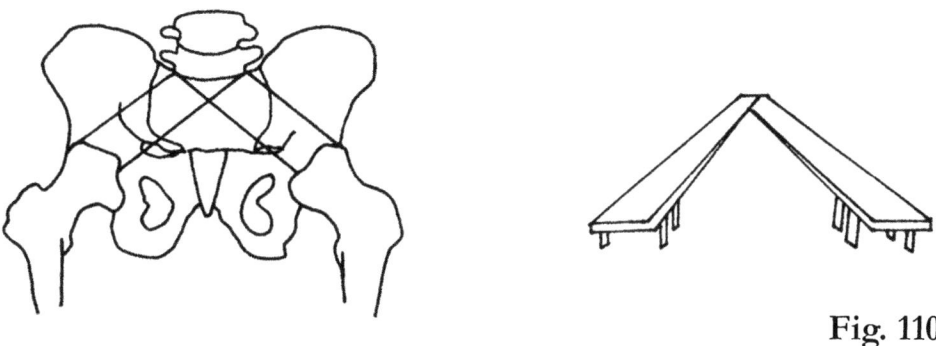

Fig. 110

In the pelvis, the two cantilevers are formed by the thick posterior arch structure of the pelvis, composed of the three upper sacral vertebrae, with the thick bone structure of the lower part of both ilium as its sides. The levers are anchored to the head of the femur by the ilio-femoral ligament. This particular set-up allows the weight of the upper body to be supported with minimal muscular effort, because the downward force at the sacral end of the cantilever is balanced by the fixed ends of the cantilevers at the head of the femurs.

The sacral keystone allows the weight, which is an aspect of the influence of gravity on the mass of the body, to move out into the pelvis and then down through the legs into the Earth as lateral thrust. This is balanced by an upward or anti-gravity effect from the pelvic cantilever structure. The whole relationship between the sacrum as a keystone and the pelvic cantilever structure anchored at the head of the femur, via the muscular attachments, is of paramount importance in maintaining the upright posture of the body. When the sacral keystone is in the correct position and the cantilever is functionally balanced left and right, you can have a truly comfortable, easy, light and lively walking action.

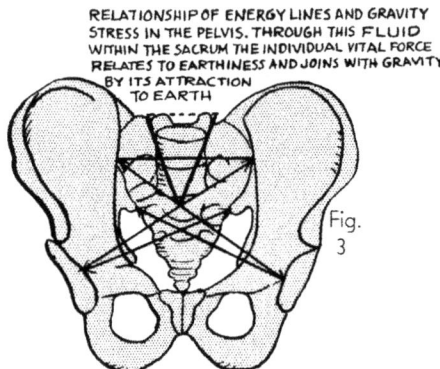

RELATIONSHIP OF ENERGY LINES AND GRAVITY STRESS IN THE PELVIS. THROUGH THIS FLUID WITHIN THE SACRUM THE INDIVIDUAL VITAL FORCE RELATES TO EARTHINESS AND JOINS WITH GRAVITY BY ITS ATTRACTION TO EARTH

Fig. 3

Fig. 111

Fig. 111 above is from Dr. Stone Vol. I. Book 2, Chart 11. In it he shows the cantilever relationship but also speaks of the cerebro-spinal fluid reservoir in the sacrum and how the sacrum is the storehouse of the individual's vital force—a reference to the *kundalini*. Making anterior-posterior contacts from the left and right sacro-iliac articulations to the opposite acetabulum, is a simple technique that addresses the positive and negative poles of the cantilever structure within the pelvis. In cases where there is significant sacro-iliac pain it is a valuable technique.

Fig. 112 shows some further relationships of the head, neck and pelvis. It shows the relationship between the occiput and the sacrum as being a diamond or kite shaped structure composed of two triangles, the upper triangle being the occiput and the lower triangle the sacrum. Dr. Stone talked of a gyroscopic balance occurring between these two bones. The lines in the figure marked 'a' show the relationship between the middle of the shoulder, sacral apex and sacro-iliac articulation on each side. Line 'b' shows the relationship between the mandibular joint with the hip joint, as well as the temporal bone

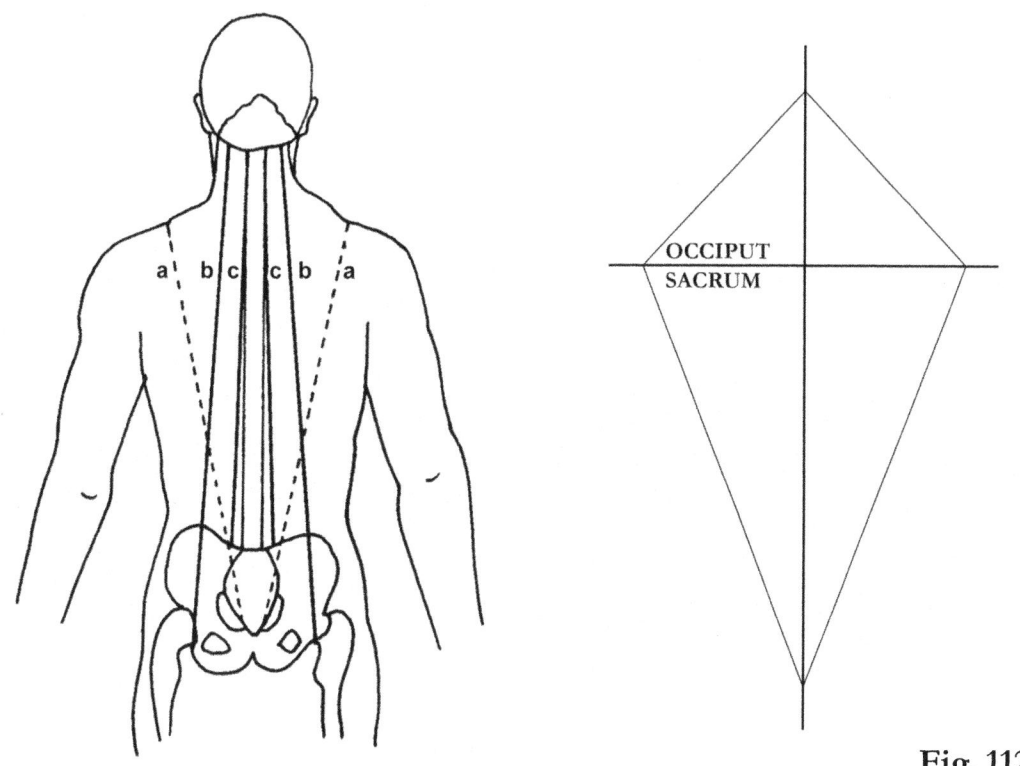

Fig. 112

with the innominate bone. Line 'c' is indicative of the relationship between the occipital base and the sacral base, which ideally, should both be horizontal.

The sacrum moves very little within the pelvis, it is bound very strongly in place by various ligaments. The sacro-iliac articulation limits the movement of the sacrum to a slight gliding rotation between the sacrum and the posterior portion of the ilium. The actual amount of movement we are talking about is a few millimeters only. However, the degree of muscular pull needed to move the sacrum out of its natural position and maintain that distortion is enormous.

As explained earlier, the language Dr. Stone used to describe the position of the sacrum refers to the position of the sacral base. He described one side as being as the *anterior inferior* sacral base, with the opposite side being the *posterior superior* side. A look at the actual boney structure of the pelvis will show that when we talk of the sacrum as moving posterior that does not literally mean that it has moved behind the restraint of the ilium. To do so would actually require many centimeters of movement to take place. When we say that one of the corners of the sacral base has moved posterior, it means that it is posterior in relation to the other side of the sacral base, which has actually moved a few millimeters anteriorly within the pelvis. This kind of posterior-anterior movement by the sacrum is accompanied by a downwards slippage or tilting of the sacrum towards the side that has moved anteriorly.

In actual practice, before trying to rebalance or reposition the sacrum, it is important to release the deep interior muscle spasm that is often holding the sacrum locked in position. This is usually best accomplished by giving the client a perineal treatment and polarising the perineal contact with the related sore points in the neck, the shoulders and the sorest spot on the back. A five pointed star release, done on the front of the body, as a final relaxation of the psoas and iliacus muscles may also be valuable. It is also useful to balance tenderness in the buttocks with tender areas on and around the shoulder blades (as per Fig. 76, p. 168).

In the five sacral techniques that follow, all use *directional contacts* in one form or another, by the use of the thumbs, fingers or heel of the palm. A general approach that Dr. Stone advocated was to pulse the work on the sacrum. He would work on the sacrum for about a minute, then let the body rest and the energy flow for another minute, before applying the technique again. He would do this four or five times. In this process, when you are letting the body and sacrum rest, it is helpful to make a satvic connection from the hand resting quietly on the sacrum to either the sacrum's negative pole (heels) or positive pole (occiput). This will facilitate the stability of the sacral correction and enhance the energetic communication between these structures.

All these sacral manipulations can be described as either sacro-iliac technique where the sacrum is moved relative to the static ilium or as ilio-sacral technique where the ilium is moved relative to the static sacrum.

Returning now to our client whose sacrum is anterior and inferior on the right side:

Technique 1

Client is on his front

1. Stand on the client's left side
2. With your left thumb contact the left side of the sacral base, the thumb pointing downwards. With your right thumb contact the apex of the sacrum, the thumb pointing diagonally towards the right hip (Fig. 113).

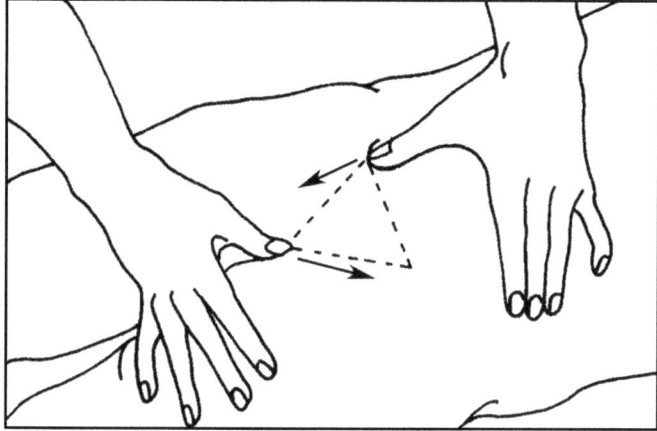

Fig. 113

3. The position of the thumbs indicates the direction of vibratory impulses to be applied to the sacrum. Simultaneously vibrate in both directions for 1-2 minutes.
4. Position the thumbs as in Fig. 114 and vibrate directionally for 1-2 minutes.

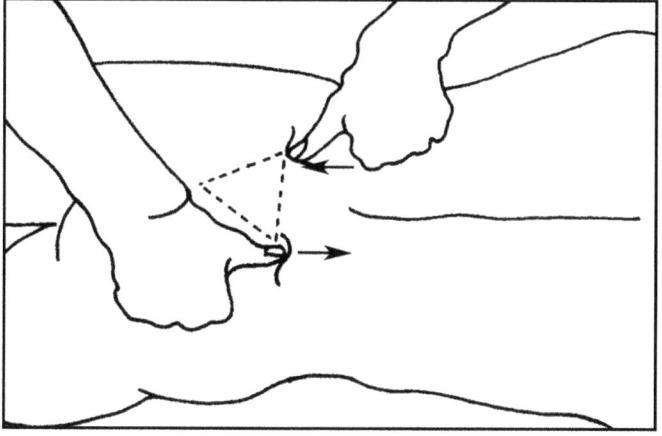

Fig. 114

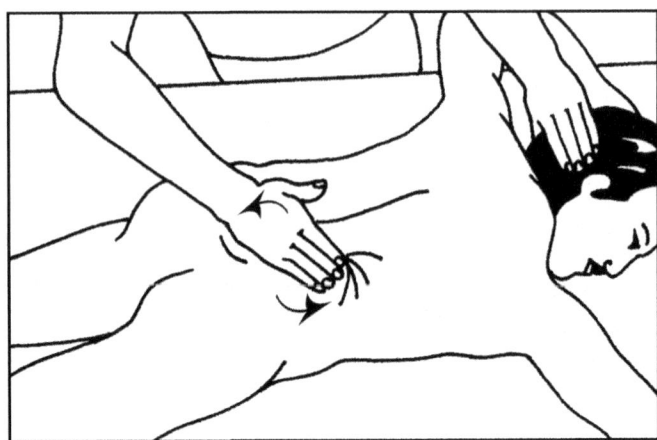

Fig. 115

5. Place the right hand over the sacrum, the fingers pointing towards the right side, and the left hand on the positive pole of the sacrum, the occipital bone (Fig. 115). Rotate the right hand anti-clockwise some 20 degrees. Apply a gentle vibration with the right hand giving the sacrum a corrective directional impulse downwards and anterior through the heel of the palm for one minute. Feel for an energetic balance in both hands.

Technique 2

Client is on their front

1. Stand on client's left side.
2. Place the right fire finger on the apex of the sacrum, palm up, and place the left fire finger on the spine of the ilium near the left sacro-iliac joint. (Fig. 116).

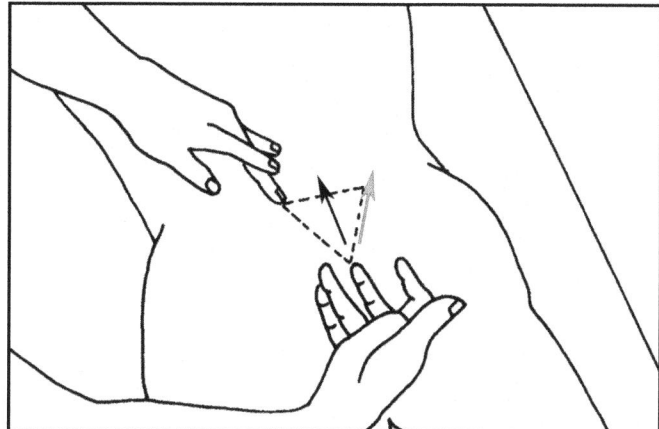

Fig. 116

3. The left fire finger is held steady, whilst the right fire finger gives a movement that is directed towards the head (black arrow) and is also lightly lifting the apex of the sacrum. Whilst the illustration shows the fire finger pointing headward, over my years of using this technique, I have personally modified it and always have the fire finger pointing to the low sacral base side, vibrating upwards in that direction (grey arrow) rather than simply headward as Dr. Stone suggested. The palm-up position of the right hand helps to remind you that the impulse on the sacrum is not anterior, which would only tend to increase the distortion. The vibratory, directional impulse is given for 1-2 minutes. The purpose of the left fire finger near the sacro-iliac articulation is to avail of the effect of a local positively charged contact to warm and relax the area thereby creating space to accommodate the movement of the sacrum.
4. Leave the right fire finger in place on the apex of the sacrum, and place the left hand on the occipital area of the head as in step 5 of technique 1. Holding the upper contact still, vibrate the sacral contact gently upwards toward the head (or the low sacral base side) for approximately one minute. Then regardless of which directional variation you use, hold both areas and feel for an energetic balance.

225

Technique 3

Client is on their left side

1. Stand behind the client and place a bolster or cushion underneath the client's left hip.
2. Contact the apex of the sacrum with the left fire finger while the right hand is on the iliac crest (Fig. 117).

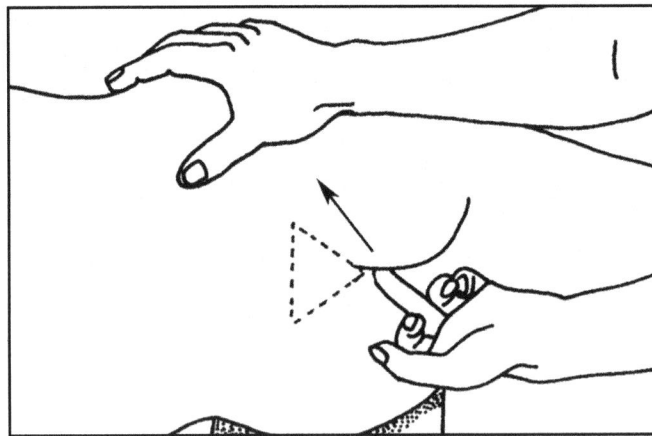

Fig. 117

3. Gently vibrate and lift the apex of the sacrum towards the right hip, (low sacral base) as you gently hold the iliac crest in an upward and towards-the-table position (this right-hand action is a slight rolling movement which opens the sacro-iliac articulation).
4. Stimulate the apex of the sacrum for 1 minute, then rest for 1 minute. Repeat this sequence 4 or 5 times.

N.B. This technique could be done with the left hand rolling the upper right ilium and the fire finger of the right hand contacting the apex of the sacrum. Energetically, this could be a superior set of contacts. You can do the technique with either set of contacts. In part, the usage of the hands above is to show the technique more clearly, for illustrative purposes, as the alternate hand position means the practitioners body is more central to the clients pelvis and would have obscured the view of the hand placement.

Technique 4

This is a powerful technique, using mechanical leverage gained from the leg movement combined with a directional impulse on the side of the sacrum. As this is such a powerful technique, you should check with the client whilst you apply it, to be certain that it is not causing pain. Generally, having the legs bent at about a 30 degree angle to the table is going to be the most comfortable for the client.

Client is on their front

1. Place a bolster or cushion under the client's lower abdomen. This helps to release the any sacral lock and lumbar tension. It also lifts sacral reflexes to the surface of the body. The placement of a cushion in this position is useful in any sacral correction when the client is lying face down.
2. Stand at the client's right side.
3. With your left arm bend the client's legs until they are between 30 and 45 degrees to

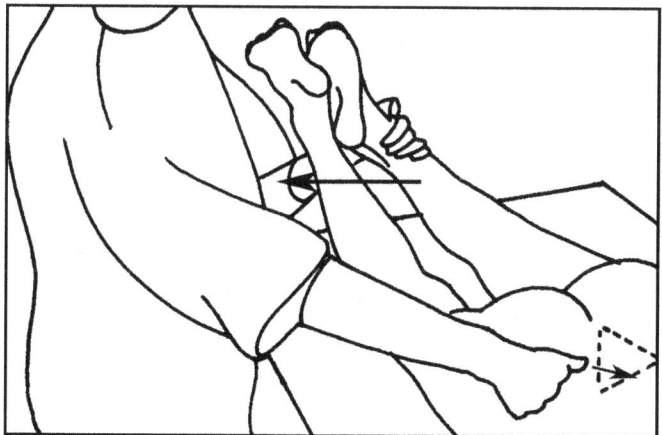

Fig. 118

the table. With the thumb of the right hand support the lower right side of the sacral triangle, at the inferolateral angle, in an upward direction toward the left hip.(Fig. 118)
4. Supporting the sacrum, rock the client's legs towards you for 1-2 minutes. If their flexibility will allow, you may also fold the calves closer to the thighs than is shown.

5. The thumb contact with the right hand may be changed to a heel-of-the-palm contact (Fig. 119).

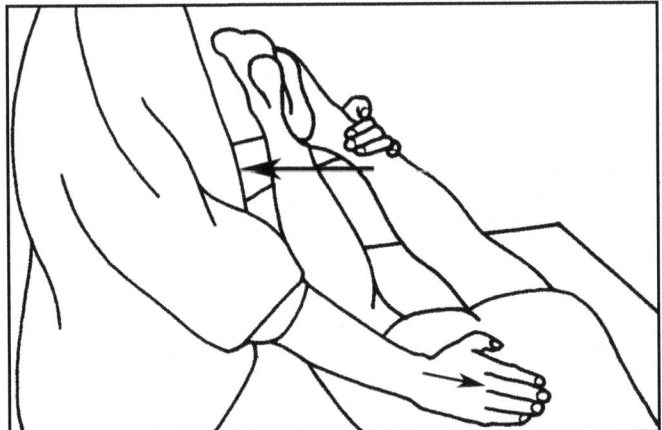

Fig. 119

N.B. Dr. Stone taught that this technique can be used on tight muscles over the ilium, as well as all the way up the back on tense spinal muscles, particularly over sympathetic and parasympathetic reaction areas on either side of the spine.

Technique 5

Dr. Stone described this technique as a manipulation of the 6-pointed star or interlaced triangles (see Fig. 81, p. 173) at its negative pole, and as such it will influence much more than the sacral position. It is useful in cases of bladder trouble, menstrual disorders, leg cramps and is also an excellent release for the sinuses.

All the previous manipulations were sacro-iliac techniques. This technique is *ilio-sacral*, in that it moves the ilium relative the sacrum, which is held statically in place through the weight of the body pressing it down onto the table.

In general, it is best to stand on the opposite side of the clients body to the anterior-inferior sacral base side when applying this manipulation.

Client is on their back

1. Stand at the client's left side.
2. Place the heel your left hand under the left-hand side of the client's symphysis pubis, and the thumb of your right hand on the superior edge of right side of the pubis.
3. Using a rocking action, the left hand is moved in an upwards direction whilst the thumb of the right hand works downwards into the contracted muscle tissues next to the bone, working all the way along the right side of the pubis. The angle of application of your contacts may be varied to facilitate the best possible release (Fig. 120).

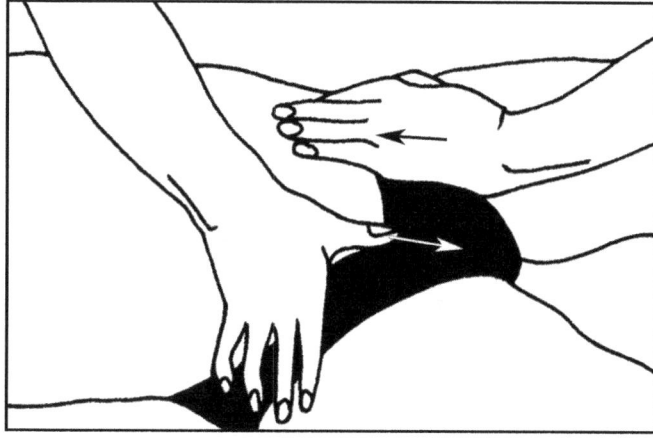

Fig. 120

4. Finally a moulding contact with both hands over the iliac crests can be made. The hands should point in opposite directions to influence the direction that you wish the pelvis to move. Simultaneously move the pelvis with directional impulses to effect a release. Fig. 121). I have found it helpful to have the image of pushing down through the short leg to make it longer, when applying this manipulation.

N.B. The illustrations are a view of this technique from the right side of the client.

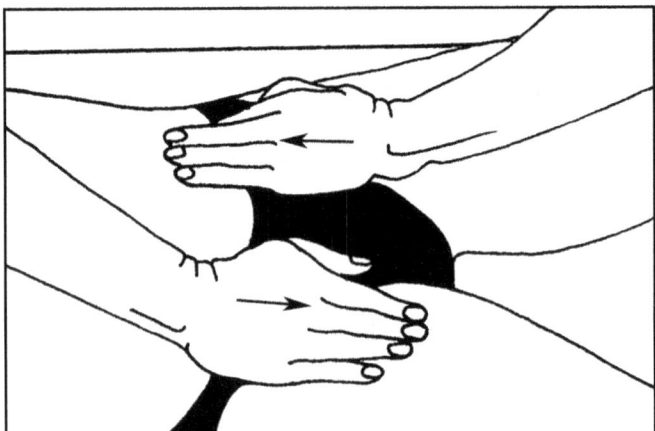

Fig. 121

Hip Correction

Having re-positioned the sacrum, you need to balance the relationship between the hip joint and the pelvis. The technique that follows is not just a hip correction but is a release of both spastic tissue and energy. The technique involves locating sore points in the gluteal muscles, and then, taking a line from the sore point through to the head of the femur, place the length of the femur along a continuation of the imaginary line that connects the two points. This gives you the line of force in giving the adjustment.

Client is on their side

1. Stand in front of the client.
2. If you find a sore spot in the mid buttock area then lining up the sore point, head of the femur and leg will be as shown in Fig. 122.

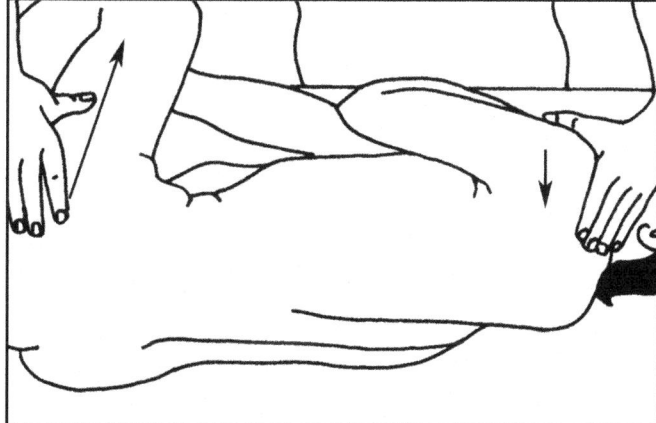

Fig. 122

3. Place your left hand on the front of the left shoulder, and hold the hip with the thumb of your right hand on the head of the femur and the fingers stretched to cover the sore point.
4. Take up the slack in the body by pushing the shoulder back and pulling down the line of the leg, giving the body a gentle stretch. Hold for a moment and then the adjustment is a half-inch pulse applied at both contact points. The direction of application is shown by the arrows in Fig. 122.

5. If you find a sore spot high up on the buttocks, the position of the leg would be similar to that shown in Fig. 123. Note that the leg is much straighter.

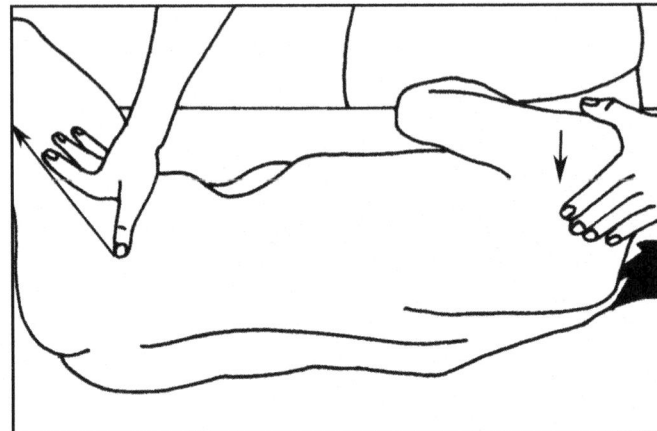

Fig. 123

6. Proceed as in steps 3 and 4. The line of application is shown in Fig. 123 by directional arrows.
7. Treat all sore spots on both sides as above.

N.B. Once again, it was easier to show the technique with the practitioner at front of the body. However, you can stand behind the client to do this technique, in which case the upper hand on the shoulder pulls toward you whilst the lower hand on the pelvis pushes away. Other than that the technique is identical.

Spinal Balancing

At this point in the structural balancing work you need to release any of the tense muscle fibres in the back that you noted in your structural ideogram or that you have marked on the client's body with a plus sign. To do this you could use a variety of approaches from connecting the perineal floor or coccyx to the tense areas, to single and double hand contacts with or against the current flow (see p. 97). Having released any tense muscles you should then check the individual vertebrae for tenderness and polarize them with all the other vertebrae with which they have a correspondence, as shown in Fig. 124.

When balancing sore vertebrae, it would be usual to balance them only with the corresponding vertebrae that are actually showing signs of distress. However, it can be beneficial to balance all the related vertebrae, whether they are sore or not.

Dr. Stone noted that it is important to release the negative pole lock to any sore vertebra before working with the corresponding ones. This is a achieved by polarizing the sore vertebra with its reflex area on the feet. The relationship between the feet and the spinal vertebrae is shown in Fig. 125.

The relationships shown in Fig. 124 are structural relationships, but as Dr. Stone points out, the functional effect on the physiology when sore vertebrae are balanced, is just as great. The vertebrae corresponding to the elements, as expressed through the various physiological systems, are set out in the table below:

Element	Physiological systems	Cervical Vertebrae	Dorsal Vertebrae	Lumbar Vertebrae
Ether	Circulatory	7th	1st, 2nd , 9th, 10th	
Air	Respiratory	3rd	3rd, 5th	3rd
Fire	Digestive	6th	4th, 8th,12th	4th
Water	Glandular	4th	3rd	5th
Earth	Eliminative	5th	6th,7th, 11th	1st, 2nd

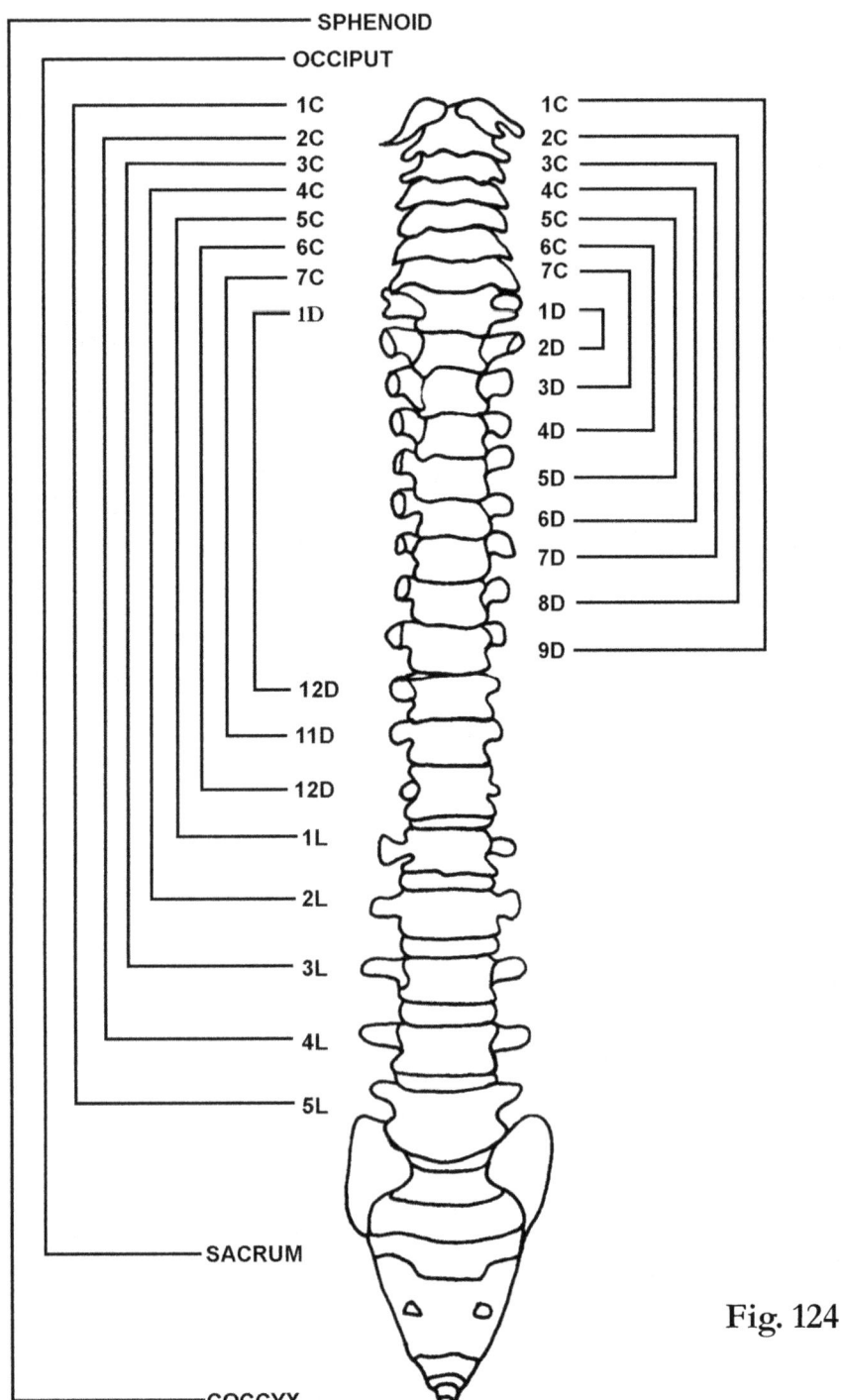

SPHENOID
OCCIPUT
1C   1C
2C   2C
3C   3C
4C   4C
5C   5C
6C   6C
7C   7C
1D   1D
    2D
    3D
    4D
    5D
    6D
    7D
    8D
    9D
12D
11D
12D
1L
2L
3L
4L
5L
SACRUM
COCCYX

Fig. 124

234

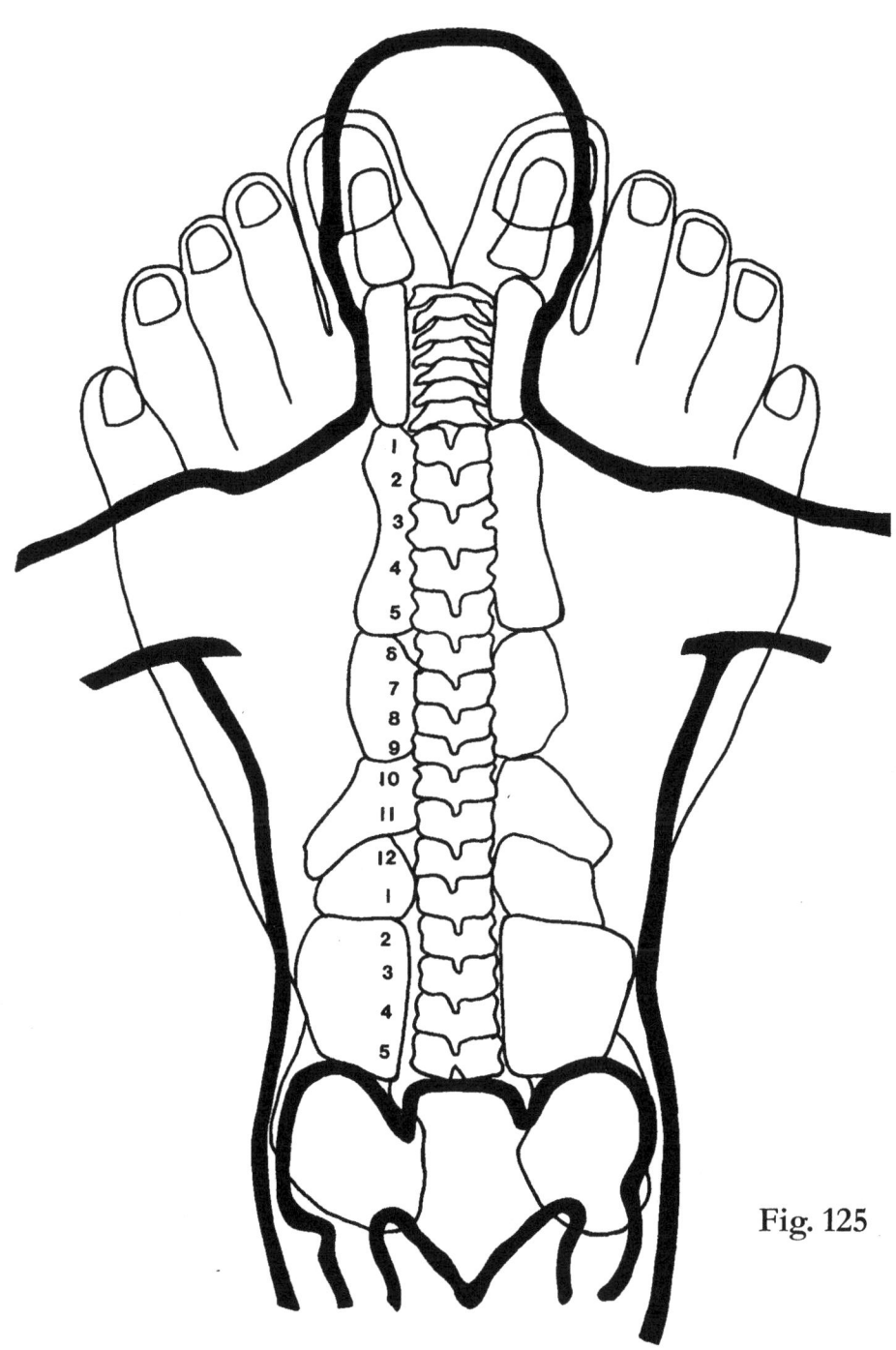

Fig. 125

Client is on their front

1. Stand at client's left side.
2. Keeping the left hand higher on the spine use the tips of the thumb and air fingers to contact the transverse processes of the vertebrae immediately above and below the vertebra to be balanced (Fig. 126). Alternatively, you may use the tip of the thumb and second knuckle of the air finger as contacts (Fig. 127). Stimulate alternately for 1–2 minutes or longer until the tenderness is gone.

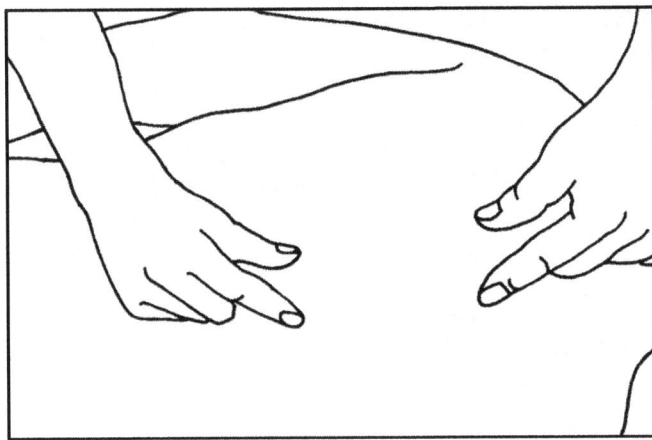

Fig. 126

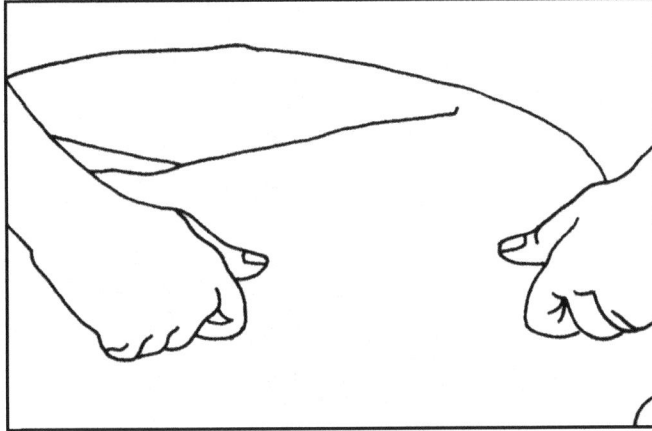

Fig. 127

Upper Body Corrections

Having released the os calcis, the short leg side, the sacrum, the hips, the back muscles and vertebrae, you now need to make some final corrections on the relationship of the head to shoulders and pelvis. The freedom of the diaphragm is critical in structural work —if it is not free now, release it! Fig. 18, p. 86 shows various cranial relationships. An important one, in relation to structural work, is the relationship of the temporal bone and its mastoid process to the back of the shoulder and the iliac crest.

Our client still has a contracted left side, but interestingly the high shoulder side has changed and is now also on the left side, so we would treat as follows:

Mastoid - Shoulder Release

Client is on their front

1. Stand at the client's head.
2. Turn their head to the high shoulder side, in this case the left.
3. Place your left hand behind the left ear over the temporal bone and occipital base. The air, fire and water fingers fit neatly over this area. Place your right hand over the left scapula (Fig. 128).

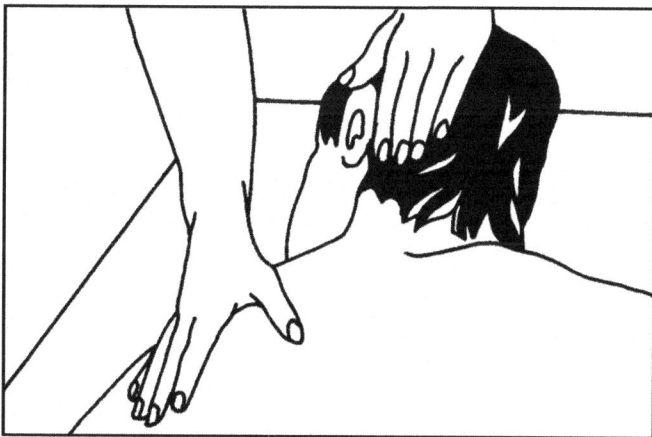

Fig. 128

4. Apply a gentle stretch to the tissues by pushing gently down with the right hand as you gently pull the left hand towards you. This is a straight line stretch. Do not rotate the head as this tends to cause spasm in the neck muscles.
5. The right hand contact may be moved higher or lower over the shoulder area and close into the dorsal vertebrae on that side if indicated.

Mastoid - Hip Release

This manipulation is useful when there is a sense of contraction on one side of the body, and in this situation it is done as an opening and releasing stretch.

The technique can also be used in a general sense for cases of ear trouble and as a release for the hips, as the parietal and temporal bones have a powerful relationship to the innominates through symmetry of form.

Client is on their front

1. Stand at the client's head.
2. Place the air, fire and water fingers of your left hand over the temporal bone and occipital base, and your right hand on the left innominate bone (Fig. 129).

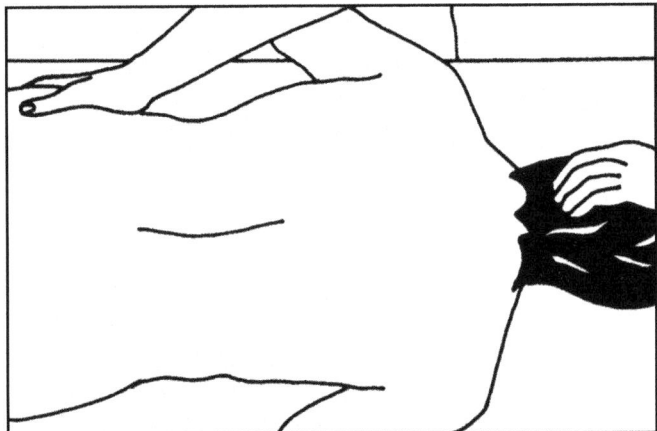

Fig. 129

3. Apply a slight stretch between your contacts and hold for 1 minute. If you feel stimulation is necessary then vibrate your contacts.

Sacral–Occipital Balancing

Sacral–occipital balancing can be done earlier in a structural session, usually after you have finished working on re–positioning the sacrum. However, it can be important to re-visit this balance at the end of a structural session. The release of all structures that lie between these two bones, will create a clear the channel of communication between them, greatly enhancing the stability of any balance you finally establish. Fig. 112 shows the direct relationship between the occiput and sacrum.

Client is on their front

1. Stand at the client's left side.
2. With the thumb of your left hand find sore spots on either side of the occiput, and with your right thumb find related sore spots on the sacrum. Remember the energy blocks often relate diagonally. Sore spots on the left side of the occiput may reflex to sore points on the right side of the sacrum (Fig. 130).

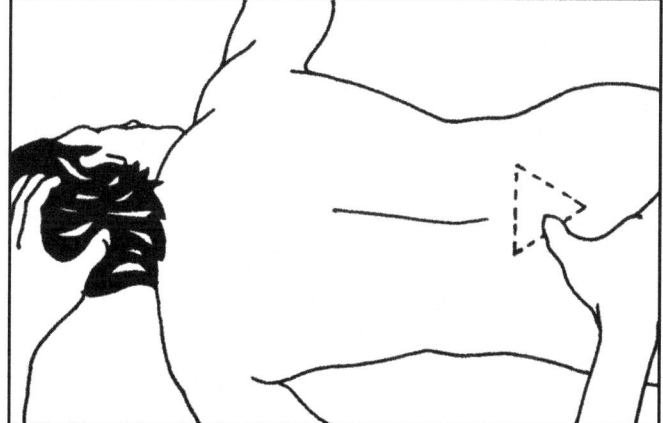

Fig. 130

3. Stimulate alternately for 1–2 minutes until the soreness disappears.
4. Place your left thumb on a sore spot over the occiput and place the thumb of your right hand on the apex of the sacrum, with fingers relaxed on the buttock (Fig. 131 overleaf).
5. Apply a gentle lift, and hold with your right thumb on the apex of the sacrum directed towards the right hip as you hold the sore spot with your left thumb.
6. Hold for 1–2 minutes. Feel for a sense of the energy coming in to balance, or it singing in harmony, to use a musical metaphor.

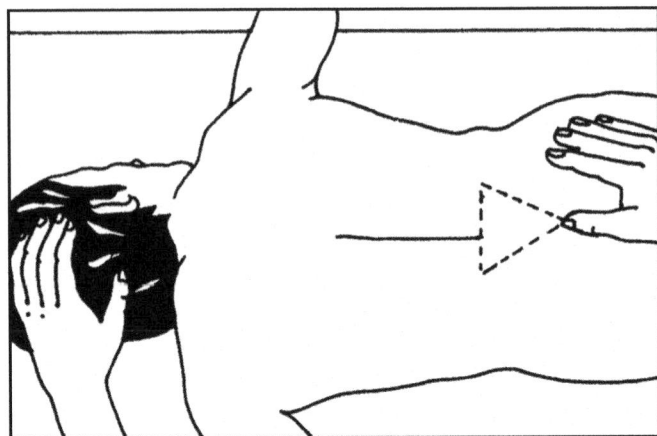

Fig. 131

7. Place your left hand palm down on the occiput, and your right hand palm down over the sacrum (Fig. 132).

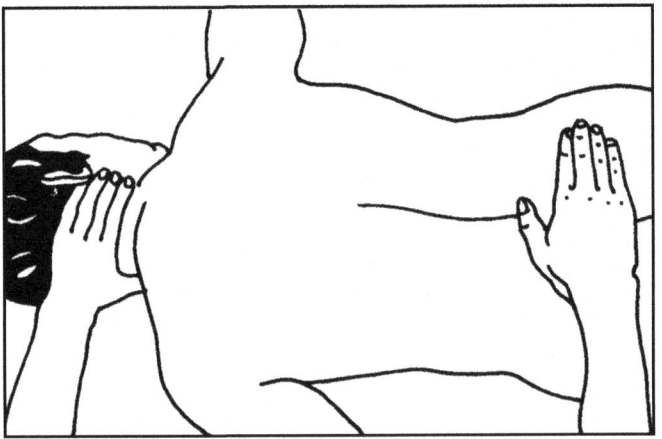

Fig. 132

8. Alternately stimulate the sacrum and occiput by very gentle vibration of your hands for about one minute. Hold and visualize the two bases leveling and balancing in relation to each other.

N.B. The visualization that I use for this is based upon the kite illustration of the sacral–occipital relationship as shown in Fig. 112. I visualize, in my mind's eye, the two bones as triangles whose bases are offset in relation to each other. As I hold and balance I see them moving into a perfect relationship, bases matching exactly, creating the diamond or kite shape of normal functioning. I find this image a powerful focus for my intentionality.

Sphenoid–Coccyx Balancing

The sphenoid and coccyx are the two bones at either end of the spine. Their relationship is shown in Fig. 124. They are, respectively, the positive and negative poles of the spine and of the sympathetic branch of the autonomic nervous system. The sphenoid is a predominantly internal bone in the skull but it has two wings that lie on either side of the head near the temples, and it can also be influenced at the bridge of the nose as part of it runs behind the eyes. Due to the involvement of the deep diagonal currents of energy in this technique, when balancing the left side of the coccyx you correlate it to the right wing of the sphenoid, and vice versa, or polarize the tip of the coccyx to the bridge of the nose.

Client is on their front

1. Stand at the client's left side.
2. Place the tip of your right fire finger on the left side of the client's coccyx and your left thumb on the right wing of the sphenoid, the fingers relaxed on the head or spread up and out like an aerial (Fig. 133).

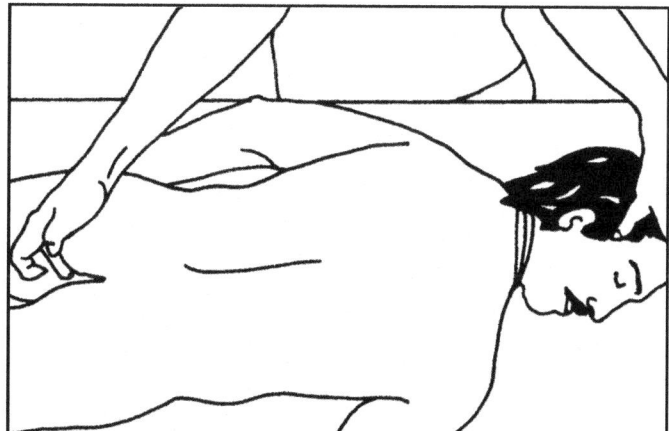

Fig. 133

3. Stimulate the coccyx gently with a small circular movement as you hold the sphenoid for about 1 minute. Hold and feel for the energy coming into balance.

4. Alternatively you may place your fire finger on the tip of the coccyx and your left thumb on the bridge of the nose (Fig. 134). Stimulate as in step 3.

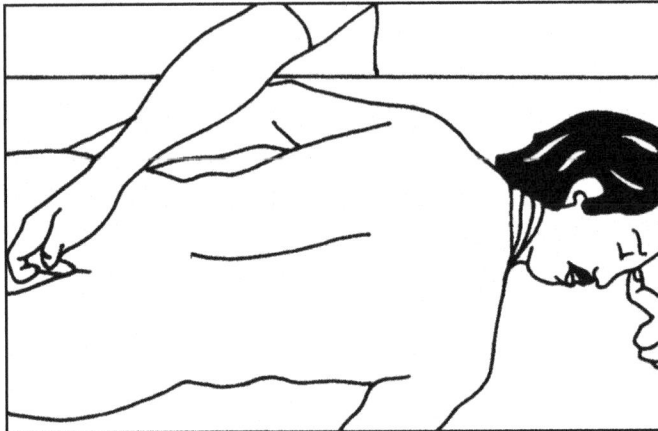

Fig. 134

The North Pole Stretch

This is a technique that is used to correct anterior vertebral curves and compression of the discs in the cervical and upper dorsal regions. It may be necessary to place cushions underneath the head and under the hips to correct any anteriority of the vertebrae before making this correction. The manipulation is done slowly and carefully. The client's body should be able to move freely on the table. This technique is not used on clients who have a long or loose neck. The technique can also cause momentary dizziness particularly in cases of poor circulation, as the body adjusts to the increased circulation of blood and energy through the neck and head.

Client is on their back

1. Stand at the client's head.
2. Place both hands behind the head so that you are holding the occipital bone with your fire and air fingers. The hand position is shown in Fig. 135. The thumbs are placed along the line of the jaw to firm the hold.

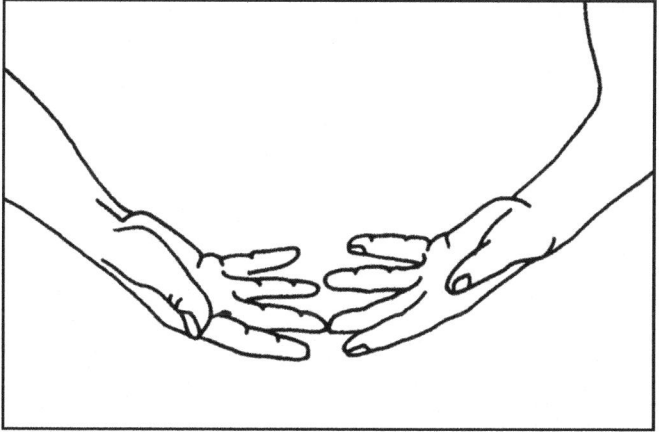

Fig. 135

3. Tilt the chin towards the chest and have the client take a deep breath as you hold the head under very slight traction. Have the client take at least three deep breaths. Allow time for a relaxation between each breath (Fig. 136 overleaf).
4. At the end of the last out–breath, provided no pain or discomfort has been experienced by the client, a short corrective pull of ½ inch (1 cm) may be given if deemed necessary.

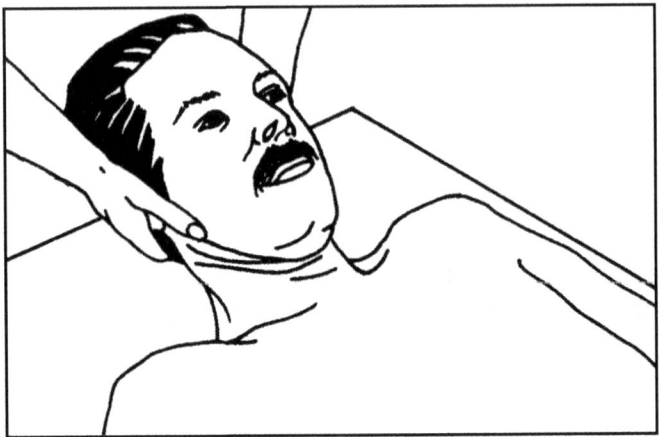

Fig. 136

Client - Summary

After three sessions of structural bodywork incorporating all of the above techniques and other general balancing as well, the main changes in our client, from below upward, are:

The heels are better balanced.

The sacrum is still not level.

The tension in the left buttock is gone.

The innominates are only slightly uneven.

The shoulders are level and the arms are hanging more evenly.

However, the major change is that the spine is now compensating naturally for the sacral distortion in that it now has a curvature to the right. What this means is that a layer of compensation has been removed.

The client no longer has the pain in the sacrum, though from a structural point of view only the first layer of imbalance has been dealt with. Further improvement is definitely possible and will no doubt occur in subsequent sessions.

10. Self Help

In Polarity Therapy the term 'self help' refers to that aspect of the therapy which the client does for themselves outside of the treatment room. It is usually taken to consist of Polarity Yoga exercises and dietary changes. All Polarity therapists should have an understanding and ability to teach clients appropriate exercises and useful dietary reforms. However, it is unlikely that any therapist could be said to be equally skilled in all of the four areas of therapeutic intervention used in Polarity Therapy. Most therapists will, apart from the bodywork, specialize in at most two of the other three areas, though they will be competent in all. My own work is mainly focused around bodywork, counselling and exercise. I do very little dietary therapy, just the occasional purifying programme and some other simple changes at most. Another area of self help is to teach the client specific energy balancing manipulations.

The Success Principle

Earlier, I spoke about the concept of never giving a client an instruction to do something that they could possible fail at. Nowhere is this more important than when it comes to getting the client to help themselves through exercise and diet. I noticed very early on in my practice that clients will do simple, easy and pleasurable exercise for years but give up on strenuous ones. Simple dietary reform was always easier than major change.

Another way of talking about this is as a *success principle*. The idea is simply to build upon success. The only way to guarantee success is to follow the model every child uses in developing their movement capabilities. Simply put, this means taking small steps and building upon that success. It also means being curious and playful.

Polarity Yoga

Polarity Yoga exercise is a huge area of practice. The subject really warrants a whole book in itself. I am going to confine myself to some generalized observations concerning its usage. One of the first things I realized after beginning to practice as a Polarity therapist was that few clients want to spend any great length of time working on themselves. The basic attitude was to the effect that I will do it for a while if it helps but I really just want to get on with life again and not be bothered about this stuff. It can be difficult to educate clients to the need for self maintenance. Polarity Yoga, fortunately, is effective when done for only a few minutes a day, though obviously the results are better if done for longer than this. Overall the biggest problem is to persuade the client of the need to warm up properly before trying the actual exercises. There is something of a tradition in the West of throwing yourself into an exercise programme without adequate preparation, exhausting and possibly injuring yourself in the first session and then giving up on the whole thing. If you are going to teach Polarity Yoga it is important to understand how to warm up and relax the muscle groups used in a particular exercise.

It is also vitally important to instill in the client the concept of 'mindful' exercise. Whilst many of the Polarity Yoga exercises are very dynamic they should never be done without a full body awareness. Without this it is so easy to injure yourself. I have a background of many years of experience both of Western calisthenics and Oriental martial arts. Through these activities, in particular the Chinese internal martial arts, I learned a great deal about people's attitudes to exercise, how to warm up the body before exercising and the concepts of effortlessness and mindfulness in relation to physical activity. I have always tried to teach the Polarity Yoga exercises with an emphasis on making the movements both effortless and mindful. One of the best ways to get these points across is in a group situation by teaching a Polarity Yoga exercise class. In such a class you can teach warm-ups, movement concepts and actual exercises with quite a different quality from that which occurs if you do it in an actual therapy session. The group situation is somehow less of a problem for people, in as much as they get to see that there is nothing unique in their inability to do some of the Polarity Yoga exercises. Psychologically this is a valuable experience in terms of their self image.

It is also important to realize that some of the Polarity Yoga exercises are extremely difficult to do, particularly if a client has led a very sedentary life style. For example, in this sort of scenario it is very unlikely that a client would be able to get their feet flat on the floor in the squatting position. This kind of difficulty is often due to tension in the muscles surrounding the hip and ankle joints. It can require a long period of gentle stretching and muscle activation before a full squat is possible, in which case teaching simple variations of the squat is valuable, as is showing how to use aids to facilitate the attainment of the position. Putting a number of heavy books underneath the heels is one of the simplest aids to doing the squat. If it is practiced on a daily basis the thickness of the books can be reduced every week or so as the flexibility increases until the feet are finally flat on the floor. Do not let your clients force themselves in to the final position in any exercise if doing so causes any discomfort other than a sense of stretch in the tissues. Pain is a contra-indication in any exercise. It is an invitation to serious injury.

There is a great deal of room for creative modification of the classic Polarity Yoga exercises as systemized by Dr. Stone. One area that is certainly worthy of a great deal of thought is that of combining the exercises into flowing sequences of movement that perhaps move through the cycle of the elements or through the structure of the body in a sequential fashion. It would not seem to be beyond the bounds of possibility to create some hand mudras to go with the movement sequences, made up of gestures that are, in fact, reflex release techniques.

Now, in 2017, I tend to work with a meta-level of exercise. I call this level simply *movement*. Any form of exercise is a specific sub-set of the larger concept that is movement. We all move every day. Life is movement. Energy is movement. As Moshe Feldenkrais once said, "without movement, life is unthinkable." Rather than suggesting clients do certain exercises, I now explore how much and in what way movement is a part of their life. I then make small simple suggestions for change. Movement implies change. Change in your orientation in space and potentially a change in locale. I work with them on changing the way movement manifests in their life. This can range from such tiny things as re-arrangements of their kitchen appliances and utensils, so that everyday movements performed in the kitchen take on new ranges and activate their muscles and joints in different ways. It can take in changes in the position of favourite chairs in the living room, as well as moving the television or computer screen to a different position. I might even suggest sleeping on the opposite side of the bed. How they move at work is another area to explore. Something as simple as getting a dog can radically alter a person's movement experience. Dogs love to move! They need, even demand regular exercise and, of course, you can pose the question are you exercising the dog or is the dog exercising you?

It is fascinating how much clients can resist such simple changes in their routine. Human beings are fundamentally creatures of habit. When people move house they very quickly decide upon where to put things and barring some major renovation of their home will never again look at the choices they made in those first few hours and days. When getting a new job, you plan your route to work, perhaps experimenting with one or two variables in terms of the roads you take or the mode of transport you use in the first week, and never re-visit these decisions again. Yet, in the meantime, over the years, a new road may have been built, bicycle paths created or a new train service brought into operation. A large part of my exploration of movement with my clients is based upon looking at the simple decisions they have made in the past and encouraging extensive re-evaluation. I use the principles of rajas and tamas, through the use of humour and confrontation, in equal measure.

I then move on to floor work and what I mean by this is that I encourage clients to sit on the floor as much as possible. One thing that distinguishes youth from old age is how much time a person spends on the floor. As a child, and even into your teens, being on the floor was a major part of your movement experience. You read books, did your homework, watched tv and played games on the floor. As a child the floor was your friend but as an adult, and in to old age, the floor gradually becomes your enemy. Re-creating that childhood relationship with the floor is incredibly valuable. In terms of movement, this simple process will allow you to re-experience gravity and learn once more how to co-operate with this ever-present force. You will begin to re-build strength in your legs and refine whole body co-ordination as you re-learn how to get down to the floor and stand vertical again.

Once I have completed this process I will then begin working with specific movements but at a very basic level. This may be as simple as encouraging a client to bend their leg and massage their feet for just one minute each once a day as they watch tv or a movie on whatever technology they happen to use. I might suggest some simple stretches of arm or shoulder that would then lead on to simple arm and torso swinging exercises.

What I would say is that all this is very client dependent. I really need to understand at a very profound level the client's relationship to movement before I suggest any specifics. What will work for one client will not work for another.

Diet

When working with a client on dietary changes the main point to bear in mind is the kind of mental emotional attachment that people can get to food. In many cases it has come to mean far more to the client than simple body sustenance, and the emotional satisfaction of fulfilling a basic need with a good meal. It often becomes a substitute for emotional nourishment, due to their inability to form stable intimate relationships or as a way of dealing with their feelings and emotions through the energetic changes that eating creates. Fundamentally, eating diverts your fire energy to your digestive system so people who eat too much are often suppressing their vitality, sometimes because they have a basic inability to focus their energy in any particular direction. I have found that getting a client to fast, for as little as one day, is an excellent way of highlighting the particular emotional reactions that they have to food.

I suspect that few people have a balanced attitude towards their diet. Virtually every popular magazine or newspaper has at sometime or another run a nutritional advice column or a series on nutrition and diet. The problem is that all the so-called experts disagree. It is also true that at any time during the year you will find a book on diet and nutrition in the best sellers list. High fibre diets have been 'in,' raw food diets, Beverly Hills diets, vegan diets, blood type diets, Atkins diets, bulletproof diets, anti-cellulite diets, the list is endless and ultimately most, if not all, of these diets are unbalanced in some way or another. The truth is, any change in your diet will produce some kind of change in your body which is initially beneficial. It is when people stick to them rigidly that problems occur. I believe there is an innate fundamental wisdom in the body that will tell you what kind of diet you should eat at anyone time. That same wisdom will modify it when necessary. Sadly, for most people there has to be quite a lot of mental-emotional and energetic balancing for this process to be able to function properly, due to the incredible amount of conflicting information that is constantly thrust at us.

I have worked with many clients in my practice suffering from different kinds of cancerous conditions. There has and continues to be an enormous amount written on the relationship between diet and cancer, both from the point of view of a poor diet being a causative factor and a good diet being a powerful remedial therapy. Many clients have taken this idea on board, to the extent that not only did they feel that their diet was a causative factor but they had also become truly obsessive about their new 'healthy' organic, vegan, whole food regime. I am not saying that such a diet is, in itself, anything other than beneficial in such cases, but I do question the powerful obsessive attitude that people often develop towards it as being anything other than a negative stress factor.

On the basis of these and other experiences I teach what I call the common sense approach to diet. Whilst I do not often recommend major dietary reform to clients I do spend a lot of time counselling them in relation to their attitudes about their diet. What I have found is that, firstly, the whole subject becomes less charged for the client, and secondly, that they change their diet according to their own intuitive sense of what is right for them at any particular time. I call it the commonsense approach because that is basically what it is. If you see a food product label showing that it is full of chemicals and preservatives then it does not make a lot of sense to eat it, unless you want to preserve your body for posterity! I suspect it is also true that if you have lived on a junk food diet for most of your life an instant massive change in your diet is not a good idea. It will probably make your body detoxify at a rate of knots, but in the long run my own feeling is that the time required for your body to change and learn to produce the right balance of enzymes necessary to process a totally different diet is often years rather than months or weeks.

I am also fairly certain that there are some people who are probably genetically incapable of being healthy on, for example, a vegetarian whole food diet. In fact, the genetic factor in diet is something that I have not seen explored in any depth. Anthropologically speaking, in any continental area there are usually races that are predominantly carnivorous and those who are mainly vegetarian. The indigenous Indian inhabitants of North America are a case in point. Some tribes were nomadic hunters who lived mainly on a meat diet, and some were farmers who lived mainly on grain and vegetables with a small meat supplementation. The inability of these and other races to handle the effects of alcohol is also a genetic factor in their constitution. Considering that at this stage in world history we are all quite mixed genetically, it is fascinating to realize that you can still easily spot people with a lot of Celtic or Scandinavian blood in their genetic makeup just by their body type and hair colour. It is also possible to recognize many other genetic backgrounds—yet another consideration when suggesting appropriate dietary changes—as if there were not enough already.

The other point about dietary reform is that, without doing any dietary counselling at all, clients will often spontaneously change their diets as a result of a series of energy balancing sessions. The better balance of energetic functioning seems to activate the innate wisdom of the body at a sub-conscious level. The client simply loses the urge to eat certain foods and also modifies their intake. Not that any of the aforegoing should give you the impression that you can ignore studying the dietary aspects of Polarity Therapy. There are some conditions that require fairly major dietary reform to effect a resolution, arthritis being one example. However, I do feel that there is an optimal time for introducing dietary changes. It is important to remember that there is always a fundamental stress involved in any illness, and to insist on dietary changes immediately is often to add to that stress.

Just as with exercise, I now work more with the meta level of diet which is *nourishment*. What nourishes you? What feeds you? Nourishment operates at all the various levels of soul, mind, emotions and body. I want to understand where a client is getting their nourishment from as well as where it might be lacking. In terms of the pentamirus combinations, the fire element is most active in this area as the basic physiological drive of hunger.

The famous naturopath, Dr. Bernard Jensen D.C., who studied Polarity with Dr. Stone, once said: "We have to recognise that there are many people out there who are hungry, some are hungry for music, some are hungry for colour, some are hungry for good associations and good companions, some are even hungry for a good marriage or a good job. There are a lot of hungers in this life and it isn't just a matter of food that is going to satisfy everything." I am deeply interested in both the type and quality of the all the sources of nourishment in my clients lives, as well as the degree to which they actually nourish themselves. The biblical quote: 'Man shall not live by bread alone, but by every word that proceedeth out of the mouth of God,' is relevant here, particularly when we look at what nourishes the soul.

When I deal with specific dietary reform, I always follow the success model. However, I also, as far as possible, take up the client's resistance. I am sure everyone is familiar with the resistance young children typically have to new food. This resistance is not confined to childhood. I am also sure that most people are aware that there are many taste experiences that, in the first instance were unpleasant but, with perseverance, a certain acclimatisation and later enjoyment of the taste ensued. In childhood, the taste buds are very sensitive and any new flavour can be a powerful and sometimes overwhelming stimulus. Think of your first experience of eating strong green vegetables of the brassica family, or your first mouthful of coffee or alcoholic spirit. Some people persevere and come to love these taste sensations, whilst others can have lifelong revulsion to a particular food or drink based on that first taste.

A lot of dietary therapy and reform requires that a client limits the intake of a favourite food and introduces a food that they may not really like. The way I approach this is to, as I said, take up their natural resistance.

To give a practical example, in the structural chapter, I introduced you to a client who was an achondroplasic dwarf. In general, he had a lot of muscular tension and inflammation around his joints. He asked me if there was anything he could do about it at home. I asked him if he had sugar in his tea and coffee, to which he responded that he had four teaspoons of sugar in every cup. I simply suggested that he have just three sugars, instead of four. He looked vaguely confused and then asked me what else he could do. I replied that this was all he needed to do. He looked very surprised and said he would try.

At the next session, he remarked that when he had reduced his sugar intake to just three teaspoons it did not taste the same, so he thought he might as well give up sugar altogether. He then asked if there was anything else he could do. At this stage, I could clearly build on the success of this small first step. I suggested that, as he drank a lot of coffee, he could try a coffee substitute instead, something like Barley Cup or Bambu (these drinks are based upon roasted barley and chicory). My comments to him were along these lines;

"Well you could try a coffee substitute, like Barely Cup, but there is problem. You are going to take your first sip and you are going to want to spit it out. You are going to think to yourself, 'what idiot thought this was a good substitute for coffee. It is disgusting. it tastes nothing like coffee. They must be crazy.' "

After a short pause, I continued,

"The only thing is, it is much less acidic in its reaction in your body and it will really help with the muscle pain over time, but you know Barley Cup really is quite disgusting. It is nothing like coffee. How they can sell it as a coffee substitute I will never know. I remember my first mouthful and it was just terrible."

I screwed my face up in disgust as I was saying this to him. After another short pause, I said,

"I would give it a try though."

He had looked quite surprised throughout my discourse on the relative demerits of the beverage but simply said, "Okay." At the next session, he spontaneously volunteered the following;

"You know Phil that Barely Cup is nowhere near as bad as you made out. In fact, I have almost got to the point where I look forward to the first cup of the day!"

It should be obvious from this example how I build upon success and take up a client's resistance. I build upon very small changes that anyone can achieve. When I suggest something new, I use exaggeration and mimic childlike responses to the new suggestions that I am offering to the client. In a sense, because I have taken up the child's position in relation to the suggested change or new taste experience, they cannot take the same position. They are forced into a more measured adult response.

Energy Balancing Manipulations

The other aspect of self help is to teach the client specific energy balancing manipulations that they can do on themselves. Many of the Polarity Yoga exercises incorporate specific release techniques, but to teach the client manipulations to do separately from the exercises can be of greater value, particularly if they have some difficulty in doing the basic postures. When doing energy balancing on yourself it is important to build up the energy in your hands, or in some other way stimulate the body (which is the benefit of combining manipulations with exercise) before actually applying the techniques to yourself.

To energise the hands simply rub them together vigorously stimulating both front and back, then flick the hands as if throwing off droplets of imaginary water keeping the wrists and elbows relaxed. Place the fingertips together in a praying position and then move the hands circularly in a vertical plane that draws small circles at right angles to the front of the chest. After a few moments allow the hands to come to rest and separate them slowly until they are about 5 inches or 12 centimetres apart. Then move them back and forth toward each other with a small movement of no more than 1/2 inch or 1 cm, until the unmistakable sensation of a field of life energy is experienced which is commonly felt as a sense of magnetic attraction or repulsion. At this point the hands are sufficiently energised to effectively manipulate the energy flow elsewhere in the body. It is possible to teach a client to do an enormous range of manipulations limited only by range of movement of their arms. For example, a 5-pointed star release from the right hip to left shoulder can be done by placing the right hand across onto the left shoulder and working down into the pelvic muscles near the right Poupart's ligament with the fingers of the left hand. Due to the limits of flexibility of the hand, the left hand probes into the pelvis with the hand curled so that it is palm upward. This technique works best with the knees bent and feet flat on the floor, as this favours the relaxation and release of the muscles in the pelvis. It is possible to teach a client to do nearly all the manipulations that you as a therapist perform on the front and sides of the body, from nine zone reflex release work to the perineal treatment. Techniques done on the back of the body can be taught with certain modifications, such as using the back of the hand instead of the palm and applying them whilst lying on the side instead of face up. The simplest way to learn how to teach these is to practice them on yourself.

A very simple exercise that can be done as the hands are placed in different positions on the body is to lie face up on the floor with the legs apart, and rotate them in so that the toes nearly touch and then out again repeatedly to a comfortable rhythm that is easy to maintain. This effectively activates the 5 bi-lateral long line currents of energy and the pelvic energy, in particular the sacrum which then through the 6-pointed star stimulates the head and thereby all the major poles of the body. For example, another version of the 5-pointed star release can be done by placing the hands palm down as described earlier whilst moving the legs for a couple of minutes, and then relaxing and feeling for the energy release. Many other techniques can be done in this way with the leg action stimulating the energy and the hands directing and balancing it.

You can teach your clients to do either specific manipulations that will support the treatments that you are giving them, or more general balancing techniques. I have noticed that some clients actually prefer doing this kind of work because it is easier than Polarity Yoga exercise.

Homework

A final aspect of self help that I use is the concept of 'homework.' All self help is in a sense work done at home, but what I mean in this instance by homework is getting an agreement from the client to do certain things outside of the diet, exercise and energy balancing areas. The kind of things I am talking about range from getting a client to do one self-indulgent act every week, to visiting the grave of a deceased relative. My own belief in the value of this kind of work comes from my own personal experience. Many years ago, when I was ten years old, my parents separated and I had no further contact with my father for some eight years. At this point I made the decision to go and visit him to say, "In case you are interested, I am your son." One week before I was due to go and visit him the news reached me that he had died of liver failure due to alcoholism. This left me with a great deal of unfinished business. I felt full of anger and grief. Some ten years later, having done seemingly endless therapy on the issues with therapists who used every approach from Transactional Analysis and Gestalt to body orientated therapy, the anger and grief were still not resolved. During all the time since the funeral I had never visited his grave nor had any desire to. However, one day I happened to be in the vicinity of the churchyard where he was buried and on a whim decided to visit it. When I got there I found there was no head-stone to mark the grave, nothing to indicate that he had ever lived, which made me feel sad and tearful. After a few minutes I turned and headed back towards the car, and halfway there, literally in mid stride with one foot in the air, I froze because in that instant I knew that I had forgiven him, and all the grief and anger vanished. Now, I know it could be argued that all the therapy I had undergone had created the possibility for forgiveness to occur but the real key was the actual visit to his grave, and somehow if I had done that earlier I know the issues would have been resolved much sooner.

Since that time I have tested out the idea, when doing therapy with clients who are stuck with unresolved grief, that in some way visiting the grave is a critical action. In some cases I have even visited the grave with them. In all the cases where I have used this approach it seems to have marked a major turning point in the therapeutic work. This led me on to the whole idea of the therapeutic effect of certain actions in relation to a client's problems. A client with problems relating to their self-worth can be shifted quite dramatically by getting them to do one particular action that somehow is fundamentally meaningful and relevant to the quality of their self-image. The skill lies in ascertaining what action they need to undertake. Unfortunately, I cannot offer any real guidelines on how to choose the appropriate action. The process for me is an intuitive perception based on a deep connection with the client's mental and emotional energy.

11. Afterthoughts

Dr. Stone often compared Polarity Therapy to homoeopathy in that the basis of Polarity is 'like cures like' (similaris curantur similaris), a concept that is common to many systems of alternative medicine. In classical homeopathy, when an effective remedy is found the client continues to take the same remedy until it creates no further change in their state of health. At this point if they are not completely balanced and healthy again their whole state is re-evaluated and a new remedy prescribed. This same issue is raised when you have given a client a session that has had a great deal of impact on their energetic balance. During the next session do you, by and large, repeat the same treatment, or do you immediately follow up any new developments that have been created in their energy field?

The clearest way to illustrate this concept is to take the example of a client with an air elemental imbalance. In the first scenario, you give them whatever kind of work that you feel is appropriate to resolving the air imbalance they are manifesting. At the next session you find that the treatment you gave previously had a good effect and that the air imbalance had resolved itself, but that they are now manifesting some degree of fire disturbance, so you treat the fire imbalance in whatever fashion you deem appropriate. At the third session you find that air and fire are now clear but that some other imbalance is showing, so you treat that and so on until all the energetic imbalances are clear and the client is healthy again. This particular way of approaching treatment could simply be called 'following the blockages.' In essence you are tracking the changes and dealing with whatever arises in the moment.

In the second scenario, the client is again treated appropriately for the air imbalance; but at the second session, rather than following the blockages you give them exactly the same treatment as in the first session. You would keep repeating the same treatment for as long as it continued to create change, and only shift to treating whatever energetic imbalance was manifesting at the point that the original treatment made no difference to the client's energetic balance. You would then repeat this new treatment until it to created no further change and so on until the client was healthy. This kind of approach to treatment could be called 'repeating effective balancing.' Indeed, these two concepts can be explored during a single session. Following the blockages during a single session would mean that you would not stay with a particular balancing approach if at some point in the treatment the client suddenly began manifesting other signs. This might lead you to change your treatment, say from working with the air element to working on earth, or you could ignore the signs of earth imbalance and continue with the air treatment.

Having used both approaches over a number of years I cannot really say that one way is superior to the other, but if I had to choose I would probably go for repeating effective balancing as my overall approach. Using this particular approach does not mean I only ever do one treatment on a client. In fact, in some sense, all treatments are different even if you use exactly the same manipulations, but I am utilizing techniques which by virtue of the client's own responses has proven to be effective therapy. In following the blockages I have come to the conclusion that the human energy system is a very subtle mechanism that is quite able to give you false leads, because as energy releases it will show up a multitude of apparent blockages and disturbances as the system balances and regulates itself. It is important to bear in mind that our energy system is self-regulating and will manage to rebalance itself very well as long as you simply maintain an overall impetus.

One of the first things I do after I have given a session, is to self reflect on my feelings about it. The sort of questions I ask myself are: how clearly did I see the client's problems? was it an effective session? how relaxed was I? did I tune in to the energy as well as I could have? what did I learn? did the client learn anything? what direction should any future therapy take? was the session an enjoyable experience? The answers to these questions and many others are not as important as the process of self reflection on the issues raised. This internal process is a form of self-supervision. If you are going to learn from the experience of giving a Polarity session then there must be a period of integration, a time during which you evaluate the quality and content of the experience and allow this to modify your beliefs about and understanding of Polarity Therapy. This is essential if you are going to improve as a practitioner. Ultimately, if you do not grow and expand in your knowledge, the work you do will become rigid and it will not be long before all the heart has gone out of it.

What is Health?

One of the most interesting experiences that I have had as a Polarity therapist is that in spite of the fact that Polarity is a very powerful healing system in the physical sense, I have often treated clients who did not improve physically and yet who insisted that they felt 'healed.' Clients who were still in fact experiencing a significant degree of physical pain. The alleviation of physical pain was one of my early criteria for judging the effectiveness of my treatments. It took a number of these experiences before I realized something that is fundamental to my practice and teaching of Polarity Therapy: this is that health is neither the absence of physical or mental dis-ease nor the experience of continuous physical and mental wellbeing. Health is, in fact, all of these things. It is very simply the ability to change fluidly from one state of being to another. Health is an endless flow of changes. Most of us have a concept of health that is static. You are either healthy or sick. When the reality is healthy or sick you are still experiencing the continuum that is 'HEALTH.'

My clients' belief in a static concept of health created an interesting problem in terms of their continuing to use Polarity Therapy as a form of treatment. What their belief did was to prevent them coming to see me if they became ill again after their initial course of treatment was complete. Once their health problem had been resolved, they somehow felt that they were not supposed to get ill once more. They then experienced a strong sense of themselves as being a failure if they did, nor did it make any difference whether or not the nature of the disease was the same as the original problem. I had originally thought that they did not return to see me when they felt bad again because they saw my treatment as a failure. I only discovered the truth of the situation because my practice was in a relatively small town where I would often meet my clients casually in the street. I would naturally ask how they were. It was then I discovered that they were often still having problems but had felt unable to come and see me because they thought they were not supposed to get ill again. They felt they had failed. What this made me realise is that I really had to explore quite deeply with them their basic concept of health, and get them to see it as a state of constant change; like an energetic wave-form, there would always be highs and lows but the main thing was to simply go with the flow. If you are ill this week you probably will not feel the same in two weeks' time. You could be better or worse but ultimately all that was certain was that it was going to be different. Coming to understand and accept such a dynamic concept of health was, for most of them, a real healing in itself. They no longer had to experience the insidious fear that when they became ill it was a sentence of doom that was perhaps going to define the rest of their lives.

A shift in a client's beliefs from health as a static condition of wellbeing to health as a dynamic process of constant change is the release of an energy block in the mind. This then allows the body state to undergo a change. It is worth realizing that any belief that is fixed and does not admit or allow the possibility of change is a definite blockage to the free flow of energy in your body and your life in general. Some of my afterthoughts and reflections upon my experiences as a Polarity therapist were that clients always changed but often did not get physically better. There was always a sense that the change was in their minds, or more specifically their beliefs, which nearly always created a shift in their emotions. Sometimes this was accompanied by a change in their physical state, sometimes not. Either way it did not seem to matter to them. Many times clients have said to me: "I came here for you to sort out my body and what you have done is sort out my mind," and yet gone away perfectly happy with this as a therapeutic outcome, even though basically this was not within the confines of the therapeutic contract.

Attunement, Awareness and Choice

This ultimately led me to throw out the idea of a therapeutic contract except in its simplest form, because it seemed that neither I nor the client was able to judge what the outcome of the work we did was supposed to be. Any kind of specific contract seemed to be a form of limitation. I have considered that if I do have a contract, what it says is 'create change and trust the life energy. It always knows best.' It seemed as time went on that I did not use 'therapeutic interventions.' What happened in a session was that my energy had a relationship with the client's energy and that 'something happened.' What this was, was never clear until later, but it was always appropriate. This was the beginning of my conceptualisation of the attunement approach to Polarity Therapy. This is not to say that I advocate this as an approach to take from your very first treatments as a Polarity therapist. I think you need to start with some boundaries and goals so you can explore the vast possibilities that Polarity offers and be able to make some sense of the responses you get. My approach could be described as being intuitive, but that intuition comes from years of study, practice and synthesis. I do not see intuition as having no form or structure as its foundation—quite the opposite in fact. The better the foundation, the better the intuition.

It also happened on occasion that clients got neither any physical improvement nor any mental-emotional change, or so it seemed. At first, I took these cases as my real failures, but I then realized that these clients were getting something else that I believe to be of definite value. What they got was an increase in their awareness both of themselves and of the people around them. An awareness of the nature of their problems both physically and mentally and what was causing them. Yet they were not going to try and change the situation. You could say that they were consciously aware of their ability to make choices and that their actual considered choice was to change nothing. I had often noticed that if a client did experience a major inner change, unless they supported this with an equivalent change in the outer form of their lives the change would not hold. The dynamics of someone's state of health is intimately linked with the dynamics of their personal relationships. I had noticed in many of these cases that it was the client's current relationship that was one of the major causative factors in their problem. This factor was often openly acknowledged in the course of treatment, and yet ofttimes the client's decision was that for any number of reasons they were not prepared to initiate any changes in the relationship. This, of course, is a perfectly valid choice and the key word here is 'choice.' Choice based upon an awareness of the facts. There is also no implication in these situations that the clients' choices will not change at some point in the future. What they have gained during treatment is both awareness of themselves and an acknowledgement of their ability to choose the kind of life experiences that they have with all the implications, both positive and negative.

Referrals

It has always seemed a rather difficult question to answer in the light of all my experiences regarding the possible outcome of a series of Polarity sessions, to determine when the work was finished. Indeed, for some of my clients it seemed as though their decision was that it was never going to end. They were quite happy with the idea of having fortnightly or monthly sessions until the end of time. I personally found these clients extremely rewarding to work with, not the least because of the depth of relationship that occurred between us. This kind of scenario allows you to study the effects of Polarity Therapy on a much longer time-scale than is usual. It also allows you to practice Polarity Therapy as a preventative health care system and to do a great deal of health education. In many cases the end point of the therapy occurred when the client was finally free of pain. In other cases the situation was not nearly so clear cut and ultimately I had to rely on my own ability to recognise the point at which the therapy I was offering was not creating any further positive changes. This was not always a point of resolution for the client's problems, and so I found it essential to build up a referral system whereby a client was not left without any possibility of further change. I think it is essential in these situations to keep hope alive by giving the client a number of alternative routes forwards. It is also important to prevent the client from thinking that their problems are too difficult to resolve simply because your work with them was not fully successful. Do not be afraid to admit your limitations, particularly to yourself. Once again the need for education on the nature of health, and an unbiased overview of the many systems of alternative health care that are available, is useful.

The only real failures that I can think of from all the thousands of treatments that I have given were the treatments in which I could not connect with the energy. Sometimes this happened at the very first session, in which case the client often did not come back for another, no doubt saving us both a lot of wasted time and energy. At other times it occurred during the middle of a series of treatments, often at what I call the plateau phase in therapy. This is a place at which there is an apparent lack of progress but which in reality is probably a space for integration before new movement begins. When the therapy reaches this point it often breaks off for a while before you get a call asking for another session. A great deal of learning can take place for you as a practitioner when you feel that you have failed in some way. It is a wonderful opportunity for some deep self reflection on your own development as a therapist.

The practice of therapy should be a joyful, fulfilling experience, not a burden. If you do healing work because you feel you must, because you need to heal, or because you feel it is a spiritual obligation imposed upon you, then you are doing it for the wrong reasons entirely. It is true that most people become therapists because they have a need to be needed, because it makes them feel worthwhile as people. Thankfully, over a period of time the actual experience of being a practitioner and the reality of spending your whole working life ministering to the sick and emotionally disturbed tends to resolve the problem. At this point a practitioner either leaves the work and becomes something really fulfilling to themselves personally, like being a builder, or they continue as therapists, becoming far more effective because they have lost their attachment to the process and do it because it is both fulfilling and fun. They are no longer caught up in putting on a performance of 'caring healer' or some other related role. Some people might question the usage of the word 'fun' in relation to the practice of therapy, but in answer all I can say is, "is it really that much of a burden for you?"

Development of Art

To practice as a therapist over a period of years or even a whole lifetime requires a continuing development of your skills. Without this you will ultimately become stale and begin working by rote instead of by a dynamic everchanging process of interaction with the life energy. There is always a great deal of talk about the *healing arts*. We talk of Polarity as a healing art. Are you a practitioner of the science of Polarity Therapy or are you a master of the art of healing with life energy? It is probably true that every student of Polarity Therapy who has successfully completed a training course is a practitioner of the science of Polarity. Their heads are full of reflexes, positive and negative poles, sacral distortions, enemas and purifying diets, squats and positive thinking, causes and effects. The shift from being a practitioner to being an artist occurs at the point when you can let go of the idea of doing therapy and have the confidence to allow yourself to simply 'be' with the energy. A definition of art that I have always felt at home with is that art is the expression of the momentary perception of truth through a particular medium. The truth referred to is not necessarily a universal unchanging 'Truth,' but the truth of the artist's inner reality at a particular point in time. The medium through which we, as exponents of the art of Polarity Therapy, express our experience of truth is our presence, our energy. The shift from practitioner to artist is the transition from being earthed in the principles to allowing yourself to be carried freely by the currents of the ether. A master of the art of Polarity Therapy is someone who can take one single technique and subtly modify it to fit ten different situations, unlike the practitioner who must have ten different techniques.

In the end, it is not the system that makes the therapist but the therapist who makes the system work. No matter how good your training the shift into artistry comes when you can transcend the limitations inherent in it. For all students, the position adopted in relation to the superior knowledge and experience of their teachers is nearly always one which limits the full expression of their unique potentials. To use a well worn phrase which is none the less expressive of the truth of being a student, whatever you are studying: 'if you meet the Buddha on the road, kill him.' Having killed numerous Buddhas, I can vouch for this as an essential requirement for the true fulfillment of your therapeutic potential!

Appendix I

The Hermetic Roots of Polarity Therapy

Any detailed study of Dr. Stone's writings on Polarity Therapy will reveal the influences from Chiropractic, Osteopathy, Ayurvedic Medicine, Naturopathy and Chinese Medicine. What is perhaps not so clear is the extent to which Polarity Therapy is based upon Hermetic principles. In his books Dr. Stone mentions Hermetic philosophy and the concept of 'as above, so below,' but a look at the seven principles of Hermetic philosophy will show that Polarity could as easily be called 'Hermetic Medicine.' The seven Hermetic principles are as follows.

The Principle of Mentalism

That the universe is mental, the All is Infinite Mind which is the fundamental reality and the womb of all universes.

The Principle of Correspondence

Whatever is Below is like unto that which is Above, and whatever is Above is like unto that which is Below, to accomplish the miracles of the One.

The Principle of Vibration

Nothing rests, everything moves and vibrates.

The Principle of Polarity

Everything is dual, has poles, and pairs of opposites.

The Principle of Rhythm

Everything has its tides, its rise and fall, its peaks and troughs; its equal pendulum swings to the right and left.

The Principle of Causation

Every effect has its cause, every cause has its effect, all proceeding by Law, never by Chance.

The Principle of Gender

Everything has its Masculine and Feminine aspects.

A simple reading of these principles should convince you just how much of Polarity is based upon Hermetic principles. All are considered in some detail in Dr. Stone's writings, except perhaps the principle of rhythm in relation to energy flow in the body. This principle is certainly covered in great detail in Chinese energy theory, and so Dr. Stone must have been aware of it even if he did not write about it. Even more interesting is the fact that many of the charts are in actual fact re-drawn, modernized versions of charts created by Hermetic philosophers and alchemists of the sixteenth and seventeenth centuries.

For example, the chart reproduced opposite as Fig. 137 taken from the book *Polarity Therapy and its Triune Function* (Vol. I, Book 3) and entitled 'Chart 4. Geometric, anterior and lateral polarity reflexes,' is virtually identical to the chart (Fig. 138 overleaf) created by the English physician and alchemist Robert Fludd, during the early part of the seventeenth century. Fludd was a leading member of a group of medical mystics who believed that their work was the key to a truly universal science. If you compare the charts closely you will see that you only have to add three circles from Robert Fludd's chart to Dr. Stone's for them to be identical. In fact, looking at Robert Fludd's chart, the other relationships that it shows are specified in other places in Dr. Stone's writings as polarity relationships. For example, the circle in Fludd's chart that shows a relationship between the calves and the shoulder area is the anterior aspect of the air element triad or air principle relationship (chest, colon, calves).

Chart No. 4 *Geometric anterior and lateral polarity reflexes as potent superior and inferior contact points polarizing the superior pole with middle or inferior pole.*

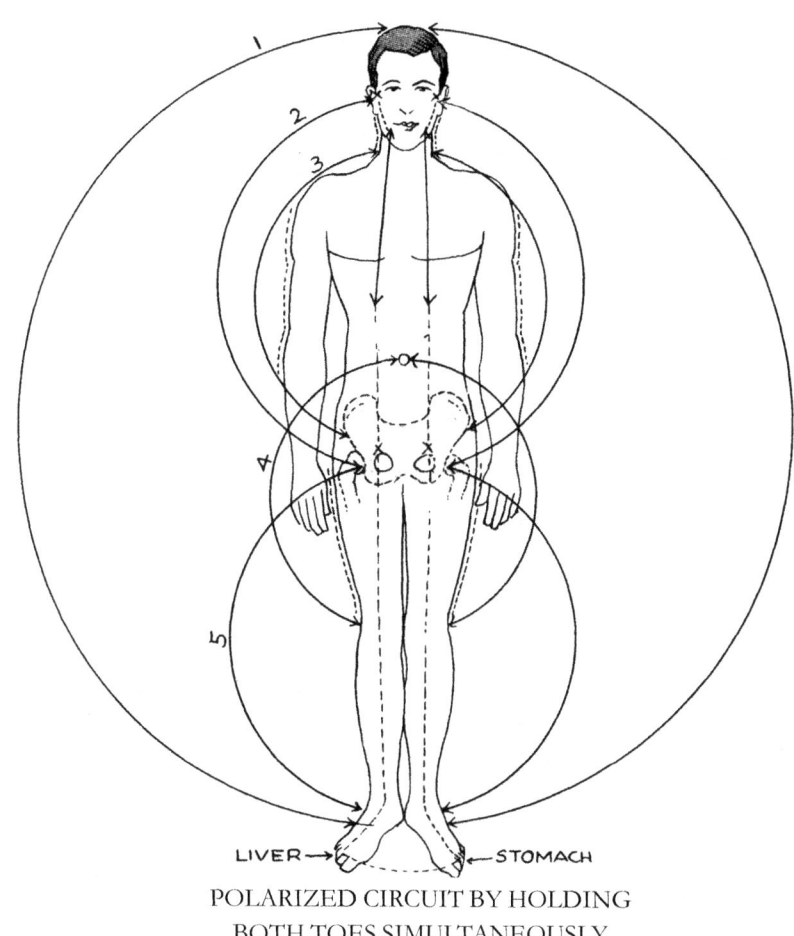

POLARIZED CIRCUIT BY HOLDING
BOTH TOES SIMULTANEOUSLY

Fig. 137

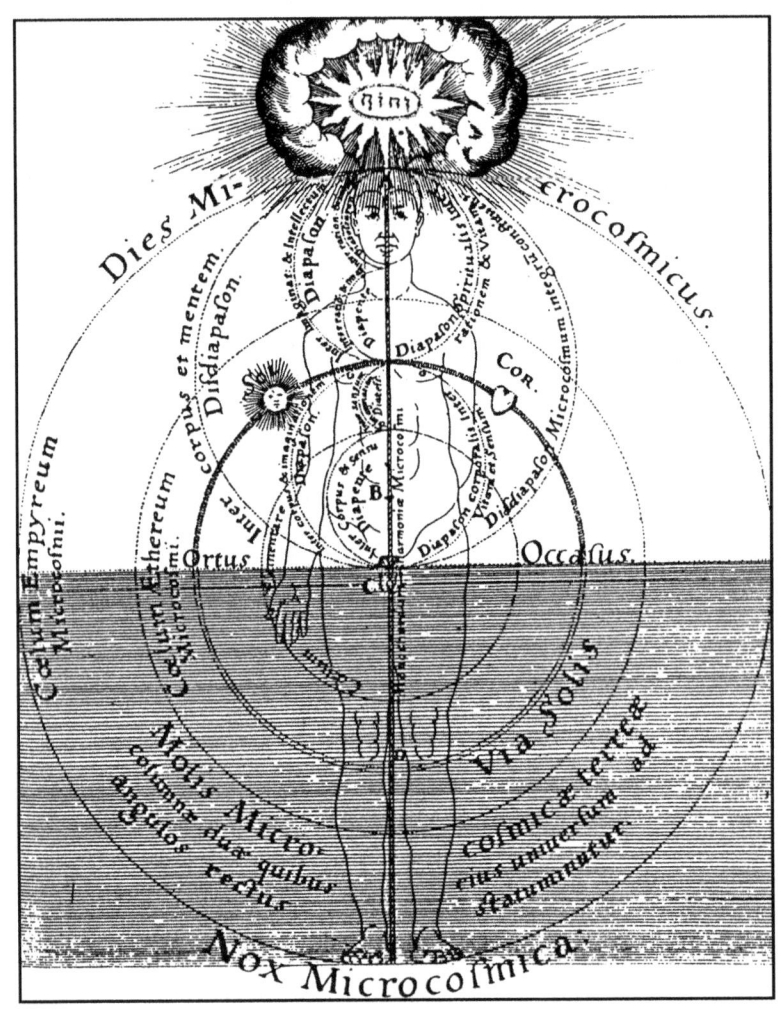

Fig. 138

Appendix II
Energy Models

It is an axiom that reality is far greater than the capabilities of our nervous system allow us to experience. The limitations of our language are also a fundamental impediment to expressing our felt sense of the subtler aspects of reality, such as the life energy. Having taught Polarity Therapy to prospective practitioners for a number of years, I am often confronted by anomalies and inconsistencies in the theory as set down by Dr. Stone in his many books and as synthesized by his successors. A guiding principle that I follow is that the map (or model) is just that and no more, or to put it another way a map is not the territory it shows or describes. Any time you work with a map or conceptual model it is essential to bear this fact in mind. If you do not then you are going to be limited by a false sense of its completeness, a feeling that it is the territory.

This kind of belief, in what is essentially just one person's perception of reality, will radically suppress your creativity. A model structures your perceptions of reality. The more complex the model you work with the less freedom for unique personal insight and creativity, except within the confines of the parameters built in to it. Most people need models because they give a feeling of confidence and security. Problems arise when the model that they have been taught has been given to them as a 'complete' one. In this situation it is common for people to confuse the model or the map for reality or the territory. The simpler the model or map that you use the greater the freedom you have to modify it in the light of your own unique experience. Models and maps provide guidelines and a focus for your intention, and very little else. A map is ultimately just a guide to help you orientate yourself when you are exploring reality. If you are not prepared to alter the map in the light of your own unique perceptions of reality, then ultimately you will find that you keep getting lost.

It became obvious upon studying Dr. Stone's writing that his conceptions of the behaviour of energy altered quite distinctly over the period from 1946-1970, during which he wrote the books and supplementary pamphlets about Polarity Therapy. He always sought to improve and deepen his understanding. For example, his ideas on the construction of the gravity board changed between the writing of *Polarity Therapy and its Triune Function* (1954) and *Vitality Balance* (1957). If you study the text in these books in detail, his concept of exactly what the gravity board showed and of the importance of structural balancing had also altered. His perception of the energetic function of the cerebro-spinal system also underwent a change between his first books, the *Evolutionary Energy Charts* (1960), and *Energy Tracing Notes and Findings* (1970). The point I am really trying to highlight here is that the Polarity model was, during Dr. Stone's lifetime, always a model in transition. It is a tribute to the flexibility of his thinking that he did change the model over a period of time in the light of new discoveries and perceptions.

So, as a student of Polarity Therapy please do not get caught up in the model. It is neither the energy nor the body.

Training in Polarity Therapy

When I travelled to San Francisco in the summer 1984 to train in Polarity Therapy, I had no idea how many students would be on the training. As it happened, there were just two of us., myself and a French Canadian man. The training was intense, focused and supremely practical. Alan Siegel, my teacher was not a theoretician, he was a practical and extremely effective healer. He gave me exactly what I wanted—a practical tool to help people. Even after more than thirty years of practice and teaching, I am still not sure of the value of deep theorisation beyond the basic underpinning concepts. To become a master Polarity therapist does not require great intellectual skills and knowledge. What you need is a *feel* for the work and to work on yourself—your own healing journey.

Ever since my own training in Polarity Therapy I have specialised in one to one apprentice style training. These trainings are unique in that they allow the emergence of the real healer within. This is something that is not easy to achieve in group trainings.

To learn more about our complete individual trainings and individual master classes in all aspects of Polarity Therapy please visit us on the web at

http://www.masterworksinternational.com

Seminars

Over the last 27 years, I have taught workshops, seminars and master classes around the world to Polarity Therapists, Physiotherapists, Osteopaths and Chiropractors. My speciality has always been sharing my understanding of Polarity's structural bodywork, honed over many decades of study and clinical work. I still enjoy sharing my unique approach to structural work. To sponsor a seminar please contact me directly on the email address below.

phily@masterworksinternational.com

PIONEERS OF MANUAL THERAPY SERIES
Volumes I - III

VOLUME I

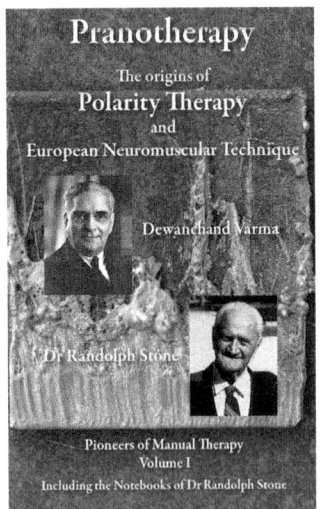

In this volume, which includes a faithful reproduction of Dewanchand Varma's original book on Pranotherapy, the reader can trace one of the early developmental branches of modern manual therapy and learn something of the eccentric life of one its early pioneers in the West. Phil Young has drawn the threads of this development together with the inclusion of the previously unpublished notebooks of another such pioneer, Dr Randolph Stone, a contemporary of Varma who, like Stanley Lief the founder of modern European Neuromuscular Technique, was influenced by Varma's work. Stone was the founder of his own system of manual therapy, which he called Polarity Therapy, and although it is similar to Varma's work, it has maintained to this day more of the original vitalistic, energy approach.
ISBN:78-0-9565803-3-7

VOLUME II

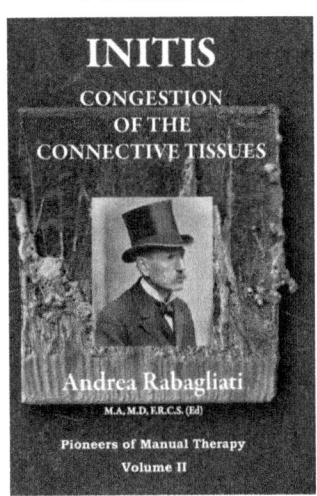

Dr Rabagliati's book "INITIS - Nutrition and Exercises" first published in 1916, is faithfully reproduced with the original photographs of his self-help exercises. The book is a delightful mix of the scientific and the esoteric, containing his unique viewpoints on the body and its ailments. His work is as valuable today as it was at the beginning of the 1900s.
ISBN: 978-0-9565803-4-4

To learn more about Varma, Stone and Rabagliati visit:
http://www.pranotherapy.com

VOLUME III

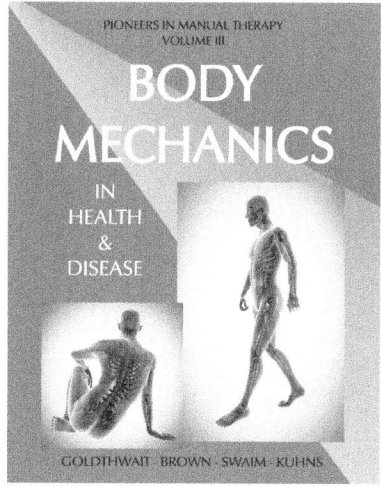

Modern medicine and many manual therapies effectively ignore the impact of posture on the health of the individual. This pioneering study by doctors back in the mid 1900s is a must read for bodyworkers everywhere. Informative and insightful, it gives credence to the importance of good body mechanics in the alleviation of many of the ailments that beset us today, including heart conditions, diabetes and arthritis.

Joel E. Goldthwait was Chief of Orthopedic Surgery in Boston in the early 1900s. He developed a successful approach to the problems of chronic diseases founded on the concept that these conditions arose because of body misalignments which in turn led to compromised organ function.
ISBN: 978-0-9933465-1-4

Polarity Therapy
Healing with Life Energy

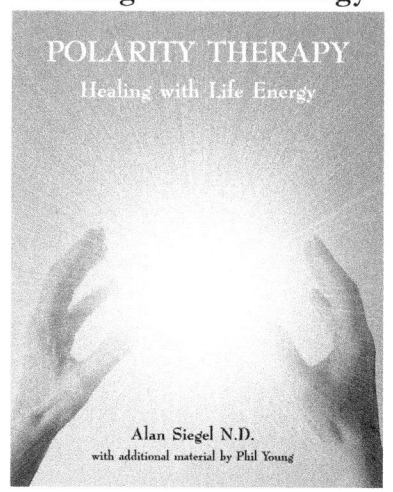

Polarity Therapy is the science of stimulating and balancing the body's life energy. When we are in a state of dis-ease or are out of balance, the flow of life energy becomes obstructed. In this heavily illustrated book you will find a complete and practical guide, to releasing blocked energy through Polarity energy balancing, nutrition, Polarity Yoga and developing positive thoughts and attitudes.

Alan Siegel M.Sc, N.D. was the former founder and director of the Polarity Center in San Francisco, California and New City, New York. He studied Polarity Therapy with the late Pierre Pannetier, successor to Dr Randolph Stone, the founder of Polarity.
ISBN: 978-0-9544450-5-8

Available at all good bookstores or online

Lightning Source UK Ltd.
Milton Keynes UK
UKOW04f2314080217

293933UK00001B/73/P